Group Treatment for Asperger Syndrome

A SOCIAL SKILLS CURRICULUM

Group Treatment for Asperger Syndrome

A SOCIAL SKILLS CURRICULUM

Lynn Adams, Ph.D., CCC-SLP

Director, Radford University Autism Center

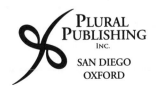

PLURAL
PUBLISHING
INC.

SAN DIEGO
OXFORD

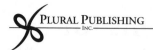

PLURAL PUBLISHING
INC.

5521 Ruffin Road
San Diego, CA 92123

London office:
49 Bath Street
Abington, Oxfordshire OK14 1 EA
London, UK OX14 1EA

e-mail: info@pluralpub.com
web site: http://www.pluralpublishing.com

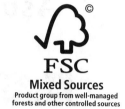

FSC
Mixed Sources
Product group from well-managed
forests and other controlled sources

Cert no. SW-COC-002283
www.fsc.org
© 1996 Forest Stewardship Council

ISBN 1-59756-022-7
Library of Congress Control Number: 2005906762

Contents

Preface

About four years ago, I began receiving more and more referrals for children diagnosed with Asperger syndrome. As a university professor and clinical supervisor, my clinical caseload is constrained by my teaching load; and I reluctantly decided to group several children with Asperger syndrome so that I could serve more children in the limited time I had. What I viewed as a compromise in scheduling resulted in this book.

It did not take long for me to realize that this group intervention idea was not a compromise, but rather afforded the children an opportunity to build social communication skills and relationships with children who were readily accepting of idiosyncrasies. Where their non-Asperger peers might not want to hear every detail of Abraham Lincoln's childhood and adolescence, in the group these children found kindred spirits. While their non-Asperger peers might have viewed them as odd, weird, and strange, in the group these children found acceptance.

Of paramount importance to me was to address the one concern expressed by all the parents of all the children with whom I work. Every mother and father just wanted their child to have friends. It is really hard to hear a mother say, "I just want my boy to have a friend." The group setting has allowed children with Asperger syndrome to make and maintain friendships. Some have joined a team for the first time because they felt more comfortable interacting in a group setting. One child decided to pursue his Bar Mitzvah after group intervention because he was no longer afraid of new people. Some of the children have experienced their first sleep-overs as a result of the relationships formed in the group. All the children have made friends.

It quickly became evident that the group sessions must be constructed to allow for the practice of many different skills, skills needed for success in school and in the world. A review of the literature revealed that children with Asperger syndrome respond to explicit rules and need to learn how to manage conversational turn taking. They need to learn how to work with others and how to deal with frustration in a socially acceptable manner. These needs, along with academic requirements, helped me develop the framework for group intervention provided in this book.

All aspects of the book, particularly the activities, have been used successfully with three different age groups currently receiving treatment in the clinical setting. Although each session should begin with a review of the rules; the order of the remaining aspects of the session can be rearranged as needed. The reader is encouraged to vary the order of the activities to encourage flexibility among group participants. The activities included in the book should be adapted, expanded, altered, adjusted, and personalized to meet the needs of the individuals the reader serves.

I hope that you find this book user-friendly, practical, and, most of all, that you use it often with children with Asperger syndrome.

Acknowledgments

The author would like to acknowledge the invaluable contribution of all the children with Asperger syndrome who allowed her to road test these activities with them. Thanks also go to the parents and student clinicians who patiently cooperated. Special thanks to Kay Alley, who collected activities as a graduate student as part of her Scottish Rite Fellowship project, and to the Scottish Rite of Virginia for their monetary support of her efforts. Thank you to Steve Mason and Media Concepts for stepping up and making the DVD that accompanies this book possible and for caring about "my kids."

CHAPTER 1

Introduction

Definition of Asperger Syndrome

Asperger syndrome (AS) has become one of the most frequently diagnosed syndromes in the United States. Estimates for the occurrence of autism range from 1 in 1000 to 6 in 1000 with regard to prevalence (Yeargin-Allsopp, Rice, Karapurkar, Doernberg, Boyle, & Murphy, 2003). With regard to Asperger syndrome, frequency of occurrence is estimated to be 1 in 500 (NICDC, n.d.).

According to the fourth edition of the *Diagnostic and Statistical Manual of Mental Disorders* (DSM-IV) (APA, 1994), the following criteria are necessary for a medical diagnosis of AS. Children must demonstrate at least one of the following:

- Marked impairment in nonverbal communicative behaviors: gaze, posture, gesture
- Lack of social or emotional reciprocity
- Failure to engage others in interests
- Failure to develop appropriate peer relationships

Additionally, at least one of the following must be noted:

- Insistence on sameness, nonfunctional routines, or rituals
- Persistent preoccupations, especially with parts of objects
- Stereotyped or repetitive motor mannerisms
- Narrow, highly focused interests

However, the DSM-IV diagnostic criteria also note that no significant delay in language or cognitive development is associated with Asperger syndrome. Cognition is indeed intact when the child is presented with concrete or literal tasks, but cognitive abilities are compromised when abstract thinking is required. Additionally, language development is *not* normal. Significant deficits in pragmatics are noted throughout the early stages of language acquisition.

Characteristics of Children with Asperger Syndrome

Asperger syndrome (AS) was described by Hans Asperger in 1944. In contrast to Kanner's definition of autism in 1943, Asperger described children who demonstrated marked and sustained social and behavioral impairment in the absence of significant cognitive or language deficits (Neisworth & Wolfe, 2005). Children with AS may have difficulty with transitions between activities, places, or events and may have a strong need for routine or "sameness." AS can result in difficulty reading nonverbal cues, and in taking the perspective of another. Children with AS are often described as clumsy, which appears to be a result of problems with body-in-space orientation (Attwood, 1998). Persons with AS have average to above average intellectual functioning, while, at the same time, being literal and having problems using language in a social context. Some children with AS are not diagnosed until late childhood; because, to most of us, they appear to be typical children. It is often only on closer examination that the social-communication deficits are identified (Moyes, 2003). Perhaps the most common areas of impairment for children with AS are social interaction, social communication, and social imagination, flexible thinking, and imaginative play (Wing & Gould, 1979). Some children with AS have difficulty with perspective taking or theory of mind and executive function.

Theory of Mind

Theory of mind involves the ability to think about other people's thinking and the ability to think about what other's think about our thinking. It involves the ability to think about what they think we think about their thinking, and so on. The term "theory of mind" was coined by Premack and Woodruff (1978, as cited by Bosacki, 2000) in an attempt to describe the ability to attribute mental states to self and others. According to theory of mind, an individual's understanding of him- or herself and others contributes to, and is restricted by, the knowledge and beliefs the individual has about the mental world (Bosacki, 2000). When a theory of mind is acquired and the individual is able to interpret the behaviors and intentions of others, the language he or she uses will be rich in epistemic or mental state words. Epistemic words are words that reflect inner conditions or internal actions in which an individual has acquired some knowledge. These terms fall into several categories, including nouns (i.e., idea, knowledge), verbs (i.e., think, believe, feel, want, hope, remember), adjectives (i.e., happy, thoughtful), and adverbs (i.e., sadly, wishfully) (Baron-Cohen, O'Riordan, Stone, Jones, & Plaisted, 1999). These epistemic words help an individual interpret his or her thought processes and the thought processes of others (Blankenship, 2000). Epistemic words are necessary to understand what other individuals think in a particular situation (Watters, 2005).

Baron-Cohen (1990) explains the use of epistemic and mental state words in a common example. Note the importance that the epistemic words play in the overall understanding of the passage.

> A man comes out of a shop and walks off down the street. About half-way down the street he suddenly stops, turns around, runs back to the shop, and goes inside. (We must understand that the man must have remembered he has left something in the shop, that he wants to retrieve it, and that he believes it will still be in the shop). The man then re-emerges from the shop, but this time he walks along slowly, scanning the ground. (Now we make the assumption that whatever he thought was in the shop was not there, and that he now believes he may have dropped it on the pavement outside) (Baron-Cohen, 1990, p. 86).

This example clearly illustrates the thought process the man went through, in addition to what an onlooker's perspective of the situation might be. The man's actions would seem unusual if we lacked the ability to understand mental state terms.

Without a theory of mind, society may seem disorganized and confusing (Baron-Cohen et al., 1999). Blankenship (2000) illustrated that epistemic words are frequently used in children's stories such as *Snow White* and *Little Red Riding Hood*. If a child does not have an understanding of epistemic terms, he or she will not be able to understand the plot of the story and cannot take the perspective of the characters. Epistemic words are integral to the successful function in daily life.

With an underdeveloped theory of mind, an individual may interpret a message literally and intended cues, such as sarcasm, are not perceived as the speaker intended. It is the listener's responsibility to interpret the verbal and nonverbal intentions of the speaker. It is the speaker's responsibility to monitor whether the intended meaning is received correctly or if a repair in the conversation is needed. When there are gaps in communication, the ability to mind read is an important aspect of effective communication and helps an individual understand social situations and to predict behavior (Watters, 2005).

Effective communication is achieved when the speaker and listener utilize a theory of mind to structure the conversation. This includes using pragmatic knowledge to organize the information to be communicated in the most useful manner. To include appropriate and nonredundant information, the speaker must remember what the listener knows about a topic. In addition, the speaker must know how to organize a series of utterances to make the discourse as comprehensible as possible (Baron-Cohen et al., 1999). Without this perspective taking, the speaker may not be able to communicate effectively. It is important to understand that children who demonstrate social-communication deficits can be significantly impaired relative to their ability to function in the primary social setting (i.e., daycare, preschool, school).

Challenges for Children with Asperger Syndrome

SOCIAL COMPETENCE

Social competence is the ability to accommodate and adapt to ongoing social situations by rapidly reading social cues. Most of us just acquire these skills, which are not generally taught. Children with AS often demonstrate difficulty when interacting with peers. They may lack an appreciation of social cues and present with socially and emotionally inappropriate behavior (Gillberg & Gillberg, 1989).

EXECUTIVE FUNCTION

Executive function refers to the higher cognitive abilities used in planning for the long term, choosing and initiating goal-directed behaviors, multitasking, and organizing. Whether a deficit in executive function is a cause or symptom of Asperger syndrome remains to be determined (Jones, 2005). Deficits in executive function can include problems in perceiving emotions, particularly when recognizing different facial expressions. Problems with imitation of another's behavior and pretend play may be the result of executive function deficits. Difficulties in planning a task as well as starting and stopping a task are attributed to problems with executive function (Cumine, Leach, & Stevenson, 1998).

FRIENDSHIP

Friendship, like many other behaviors, follows a sequence of development (Roffey, Tarrant, & Majors, 1994). In the early stages, children learn to shift from playing next to another child to playing with that child. Along with this shift comes sharing and turn-taking, skills, which often are difficult for the child with AS. The next stage in the development of friendship requires an understanding of reciprocity, the notion that friends help and support each other in order to facilitate the friendship. Children with AS may need assistance in understanding this aspect of friendship. The child may need practice with giving compliments, showing care and compassion, and helping out when necessary (Attwood, 1998).

NONVERBAL COMMUNICATION

Children with AS have difficulty reading and understanding nonverbal communication. They may not recognize and process facial expressions, sarcasm, and other prosodic patterns. They may misunderstand a joke or a conversation. This may put them at risk for ridicule and more social isolation (Adams & Earles, 2004; Earles, 2003).

VERBAL COMMUNICATION

Asperger syndrome has, as one of its reported clinical features, normal early language development. Although early syntactic and semantic development may follow a relatively normal course of development, pragmatics, or the rules of using language in a social context, are impaired in children with AS. Children with AS often have difficulty relinquishing the conversational turn, making effective eye contact, and initiating and maintaining a topic not of their choosing.

ACADEMIC ACHIEVEMENT

Although children with AS have average to above-average intellectual abilities, they often struggle academically. Deficits in central coherence may be responsible for the academic difficulties encountered by children with AS who have demonstrated IQs at least in the average range (Frith, 1989). Central coherence is the tendency to combine diverse information to construct higher level meaning, in other words, to make sense of situations and events (Cumine, Leach, & Stevenson, 1998).

SELF-MANAGEMENT

Self-management can be divided into four general categories: self-monitoring, self-assessment, self-instruction, and self-reinforcement (Loftin, 2005). Children with AS usually need direct instruction to develop self-management skills. In particular, self-regulation, the balancing of arousal, alertness, and comfort, may be problematic for children with AS. In some children, engaging in behaviors such as rocking, hand-flapping, or finger-flicking may be a means for calming and organizing to achieve self-management (Landers, 2005).

SENSORY PERCEPTION

Another important aspect of AS is difficulty with sensory processing. Sensory information coming in from the seven sensory domains (visual, auditory, gustatory, olfactory, somatosensory, vestibular, proprioceptive), if not effectively perceived, organized, and processed, may result in many of the unusual behaviors observed in children with AS (Vuletic, 2005).

MOTOR SKILLS

Children with AS have been described as clumsy (Ehlers & Gillberg, 1993; Gillberg & Gillberg, 1989). Studies have demonstrated that children with AS have difficulty with locomotion, balance, handwriting, scissor use, rhythm, and eye-hand coordination (Manjiviona & Prior, 1995). As a result of these motoric deficits, children with AS may find themselves excluded from typical play/sport activities, thus furthering their social isolation. Some possible accommodations include using a keyboard, and pairing a highly desired activity with a motor task to increase motivation. Rather excusing a child from physical education, perhaps the child with AS could be the equipment manager or keep score or write down the runner's times during races.

Group Intervention

ASPECTS OF GROUP INTERVENTION

Rules

For group intervention to be successful, several principles must be employed. First and foremost, rules for the group must be established. It is important to include children with AS in the establishment of the rules. That said, it is important to monitor the rules offered by the children. For example, one child in a group at the local university program suggested that one rule read: "No wigs in group." We discussed that this had not been a problem in the past and that we probably did not need such a rule. We did suggest that, should wigs become a problem, we would add a rule! The following is an example of the rules established by a group of children, aged 9 to 11 with AS.

Group Rules

Raise your hand before you talk.

Keep good eye contact.

Listen when others are talking.

Take turns talking about topics of interest.

Use your inside voice.

Walk in line inside the building.

Themes

Another principle that facilitates the success of the group is using themes to guide its conduct. Using themes allows for consistency from session to session and also increases the redundancy of concepts being addressed. Children with AS need repetition and redundancy to facilitate their learning. Themes used by groups in our center have included: A Trip Around the World, The Problem-Solving Olympics, Science, History, Holidays, The Secret Garden, A Day at the Beach, Books to Read, and Community Helpers.

Conversation Skills

It is imperative that opportunities for conversation be actively incorporated into the group setting. Greetings should be explicitly targeted as children with AS often fail to greet and close during social communicative exchanges. Additionally, the teacher should take baseline measures for conversational turn-taking. Once the baseline is established, the teacher can target an appropriate number of conversational turns for each child. It is important to limit the number of conversational turns for group members who tend to "lecture" on particular topics of interest. Children with AS enjoy providing information on topics that interest them but often fail to allow their conversational partner to participate in a meaningful way. Lunchtime groups are becoming popular and are reportedly quite helpful in facilitating conversational exchanges (Lord-Larson & Kaufman, 2005).

Problem Solving

A goal of every treatment session should be the inclusion of group problem-solving activities. All participants need to be included by giving each a role or item for the ultimate end project. It is desirable to have a representation of the end product available, if possible, and to encourage and facilitate collaboration as the children may want to work independently.

Games

"Sometimes we win, sometimes we lose—it is just fun to play the game." That is the mantra that is repeated during game playing. Children with AS often have a difficult time losing gracefully during simple game activities. This does not serve to foster friendships and should be a goal of nearly every session. Games can range from board games to card games.

Role-Play

Children with AS benefit from role-playing activities. Playing roles affords the child the opportunity to view situations from the perspective of others, something that may not come easily to the child. Role-playing activities can include writing a play (playwright) and acting it out (actor). The child might present book reports (book reviewer). Each child can be assigned a subject to report on (reporter), and the group can produce a newspaper (publishers). Maybe one of the children would like to be a scientist, historian, or a naturalist. Each child's unique talents and interests should be considered.

Reward System

Nothing elaborate is needed for a reward system. Stickers work for most children. Older children will collect points willingly. What is important is that an ultimate reward be agreed upon at the initiation of the group and the time period for that reward be established at that time. The group members should be encouraged to vote on the ultimate reward, which might be a party, special computer time, or even special snacks. Voting is important because it gives the children an opportunity to understand that they do not always get their chosen reward, but that the majority decides—just like in the real world.

PRINCIPLES OF GROUP INTERVENTION

Participants

Children with AS should be grouped according to their individual needs, deficits, and developmental/age levels. Including children with high-functioning autism spectrum disorder (ASD) may be beneficial for them because children with ASD are often more able linguistically and academically.

Structuring the Sessions

The following is an example of how a typical group session might be structured. Other than beginning with the sharing of personal information, the other activities can be ordered in any way that facilitates the session objectives.

1. **Sharing personal information/experiences:** This is an important part of the session as it allows participants to share information within a proscribed time period. It is important that each child's sharing time be monitored because children with AS may tend to dominate the sharing or include unrelated information.

   - Weekend activities
   - Favorite things

- Wishes
- TV/movies
- Upcoming special events

2. **Group problem solving:** This is an important part of the session because it requires children with AS to work cooperatively to solve a problem. Children with AS often prefer to work independently or attempt to control the problem-solving activity. The activity can involve building or creating something. Problem solving can also include finding a viable solution for a dilemma. It is helpful to have specific goal in mind or a picture of the end product, if appropriate. With intricate building activities it is important to have a photo or a picture to guide the group to the end product. Materials needed to complete the activity are given out by the group leader or by group members assigned this responsibility. It is vital that each group member has an integral role in completion of the activity. Members need to learn how to prompt one another appropriately for successful task completion.

3. **Group game playing:** Most children with AS do not like to lose at games and often do not lose gracefully. It is, therefore, crucial to include these types of activities in each group session. Graceful losing must be modeled for these children and using a script for games is important. The "mantra" could be, "Sometimes I win, sometimes I lose. It is just fun to play the game." This must be repeated often, and meltdowns following losses must not be indulged, but rather the mantra must be repeated and the outburst ignored.

4. **Scripting and role playing:** Social stories and scripting are vital to the development of appropriate social communication skills in children with AS. The teacher can utilize prewritten scripts or stories or develop novel scripts or stories with input from the group. With the guidance of the teacher, the group can identify situations that present challenges and script accordingly. The group can write short plays and practice social communication skills within the context of the play.

The activities described in the chapters that follow have been "road tested" in group intervention with children demonstrating Asperger syndrome. Activities that facilitate cooperative work, eye contact, and turn-taking are described in subsequent chapters. The reader is encouraged to adapt these activities as necessary for specific group needs. Activities are grouped in chapters by age. The first age group addressed in the curriculum is the preschool age group, including children between the ages of 3 and 5 years. The next chapter provides activities for children between the ages of 6 and 9 years, while the final chapter addresses the needs of children between 10 and 12 years of age. Readers are also encouraged to adapt activities described for one age group to suit the needs of other age groups.

CHAPTER 2

Activities for Children Three to Five Years of Age

Cooperative Skills

1. TRAINS

Objective

Child will use cooperative skills in a group activity.

Materials

- ☐ train track that has parts easily assembled by preschoolers
- ☐ a train-car for each child. (Push-trains only, not motorized.)
- ☐ a large sheet of paper on which the assembled train track has been traced

Procedure

Begin the session with the track disassembled into its various pieces. Lay out the paper showing the traced track, and place a piece of the track on the tracing. Explain that the children get to build the track themselves by taking turns. Hand a piece to the first child and encourage him or her to connect it to the section already placed. Continue handing out pieces one at a time to each child to connect the track until it is complete.

Next, demonstrate how a train car can be pushed along the track, imitating a train whistle and wheel chugging noises to capture the children's interest. Distribute a train car to each child and let them play with their trains on the track, moderating their actions as needed. If they recognize that their train cars can hook together and attempt to play together in that fashion, encourage cooperative play. If the size of the track or the actions of the group prohibit all the children from playing with their trains at one time, alter the train play into a turn taking activity with only two children playing on the track at a time.

2. WE ARE A TRAIN

Objective

Child will use cooperative skills in a group activity.

Materials

☐ small flat rolling platforms that can be used as "trains" (one for each person in the group)

☐ picture of a train

Note: Rolling platforms, approximately 1 square foot in size, made to hold large potted plants work great for this activity.

Procedure

Explain to the children that you are going to all work together to make a train. Show a picture of a train, pointing out how the cars follow each other along the train's path. Designate a path in the classroom that your train will follow (circling a table or other large object helps children stay on the path). Show the children how you sit on a platform, rolling it by pushing with your feet.

Line up all the "trains" together, assigning one to each child. Help each child get seated. Start the train rolling and enjoy! (Be flexible in allowing children to get "off-track" as they explore the rolling movement.)

3. RAINY DAY SINGING AND FUN

Objective

Child will use cooperative skills in a group activity.

Materials

- ☐ large paper to make a mural
- ☐ markers or paints
- ☐ rain items such as umbrella, raincoat, hat, galoshes

Procedure

Sit in a circle on the floor and sing the "What's the Weather" song to the tune of "Oh My Darlin', Clementine":

What's the Weather

(Start with hands out, palms up, as if asking a question)

What's the weather, what's the weather, what's the weather out today?

Tell me children, what's the weather, what's the weather out today?

Is it sunny? (hands over head shape circle for sun)

Is it cloudy? (hands over eyes)

Is it rainy out today? (fingers trickle down like raindrops)

Is it snowy? (shiver and hug self like cold)

Is it windy? (hands swish like wind)

What's the weather out today?

Elicit answers from the children about the weather outside today. Discuss that rain comes from the sky, and sometimes there is thunder and lightning when it rains, leading into the song, "There Is Thunder" sung to the tune of "Are You Sleeping?"

There Is Thunder

(hand patting floor)	There is thunder, there is thunder,
(hands still patting floor)	Hear it roar, hear it roar
(snapping fingers)	Pitter patter raindrops, pitter patter raindrops
(shake hands like wet)	I'm all wet, I'm all wet!

Talk about what is used when it rains: umbrella, raincoat, rain hat, galoshes. Show examples of each. Then explain that the group will make a rainy day mural depicting rain and clouds and all the items we need when it rains. Take out the large piece of paper and the markers or paints. Seat the children around the paper so that each can reach an area in which to draw or paint. Encourage the children in drawing umbrellas, raindrops, and so forth. Put the mural on prominent display when it is finished.

4. INDOOR FALL HIKE

Objective

Child will use cooperative skills in a group activity.

Materials

- ☐ pretty colored fall leaves
- ☐ bag

Procedure

Before the session, collect a generous supply of pretty fall leaves of various colors. Keep them hidden in a bag.

Instruct the group to stand in a circle. Hold the bag of leaves behind your back. Lead the group in singing, "Hiking In the Woods" (*see next page*). After the third round, stop and whisper to the group, "We have hiked deeply into the woods; around us are beautiful, tall trees; we hear the wind blow (whhhwhhh). Now everybody close your eyes" (repeat until eyes are closed) "and we'll find out what we see. When I count to '3' open your eyes—1-2-3!" On the count of 3, throw a handful of leaves into the air in the center of the circle—allow the children to scramble about gathering up leaves.

Elicit their comments about the leaves by asking questions such as: "How many do you have?" and "What colors did you get?" or "Who has a red leaf?" and so on. Finally, instruct the children to work as a group to clean up all the leaves and put them back in the bag.

Repeat according to the interest of the group. At the close of the activity, allow each child to choose a set number of leaves to take home.

Hiking in the Woods (tune: "Bringing in the Sheaves")

(All march in place while singing)

"Hiking in the woods,

Hiking in the woods,

We'll find pretty colors

Hiking in the woods—again!"

(repeat 3 times)

5. LITTLE RED HEN

Objective

Child will use cooperative skills in a group activity.

Materials

- ☐ storybook with the "Little Red Hen" story
- ☐ hats or headbands with appropriate ears to depict the animals of the story

Procedure

Read the story to the children, making sure to show the pictures of the animals. At the end of the story, tell them you are going to read it again, but this time the children get to help tell the story. Explain that you will read the part of the Little Red Hen, but you need helpers to say the other animal's part, "Not I." Demonstrate how they may shake head vigorously while responding, "Not I." Choose children to be the cat, dog, pig, and so on and give them the hats or headbands showing the ears of the animals they are portraying. Read the story again, cueing each child to respond at the appropriate times.

> *Hint:* This activity requires adaptation according to the number of children in the group. If there are more children than there are animals depicted in the book, have two or three children act together as a group of cats, dogs, or pigs who simultaneously respond "not I" at the appropriate times.

6. BALLOON HIT

Objective

Child will use cooperative skills in a group activity.

Materials

☐ large inflated balloon

Procedure

Have the children sit in a circle on the floor. Show them the balloon, demonstrating how it floats in the air but requires continuous hitting to keep it up there. Explain that the group must work together to keep the balloon from hitting the ground, but that each time they hit the balloon, they must pass it to another person. Demonstrate the illegal turn taking of keeping the balloon all to oneself. Start the balloon in the air and join in the fun. Moderate the activity as needed. Have several extra balloons on hand in case one gets popped.

Caution: Be sure to inquire if any of the children have allergies to balloons or latex prior to this activity.

7. PLATE FACES

Objective

Child will use cooperative skills in a group activity.

Materials

- ☐ paper plates
- ☐ construction paper cutouts of facial features
- ☐ pieces of yarn
- ☐ glue
- ☐ mirror

Procedure

Discuss the various parts of a face and label each cutout for each feature. Give each child all of the pieces for one feature. For example, one child gets all the eyes. Have the children ask each other for needed pieces. Encourage them to ask for pieces that closely match their own features (blue eyes, brown hair). The teacher can be responsible for gluing pieces on the plates.

Variation: Make plate faces for other family members.

---

8. SEASONS BOOK

Objective

Child will use cooperative skills in a group activity.

Materials

☐ book featuring seasons of the year with illustrations

Procedure

Discuss the four seasons and focus on the season corresponding with the current date. Read the book and lead a discussion on each season by asking simple wh-questions (What is this? What do we wear? Who has a sled?). Encourage all students' participation by directing questions to them or by eliciting comments.

9. FAVORITE THINGS COLLAGE

Objective

Child will use cooperative skills in a group activity.

Materials

- ☐ various magazine pictures of foods, toys, clothing, pets, people, and so forth
- ☐ glue
- ☐ butcher paper
- ☐ tempera paint

Procedure

Talk to the children about their favorite things, such as pizza, dogs, or race cars. Have the children choose pictures of their favorite things. The teacher should facilitate the choices and gluing of the pictures on the butcher paper.

Encourage discussion among the children of their choices to show what they have in common and how they are different. Personalize the collage by making hand prints of each child and writing their names by their handprints.

> *Caution:* Some children with AS are resistant to getting their hands dirty. Encourage participation with a reward and allow the children to wash their hands immediately.

10. APPLE-BANANA COOLER

Objective

Child will use cooperative skills in a group activity.

Materials

- ☐ blender
- ☐ paper cups
- ☐ ½ cup yogurt
- ☐ ½ cup chilled apple juice
- ☐ 1 ripe banana
- ☐ dash of cinnamon (optional)

Makes 4 servings.

Procedure

Give each child an ingredient for the cooler. Have one child acting as the head chef who asks for each ingredient. Each child places his or her item in the blender. Once all ingredients are in the blender, allow each child the chance to push the button to blend the ingredients.

Serve each child a small portion of the beverage. Encourage the children to ask for more.

Variation: Try other juices and fruits.

Eye Contact

1. TELL ME WHAT YOU FEEL

Objective

Child will use eye contact in communication.

Materials

- ☐ bag
- ☐ objects children can identify by feeling

Procedure

Gather a variety of objects. Make sure they are easily distinguishable by size, shape, or texture. Place one item in the bag and keep the others hidden elsewhere.

Instruct the children that you have something hidden in the bag. Tell them they will each have a chance to reach in the bag and feel it, and they must look at you while telling you how the "thing" feels. If a child takes his or her turn without providing you eye contact, praise the description and tell him or her to look at you and tell you again. After all of the children have felt the item, reveal its identity by showing the object; then start with a new object.

> *Hint:* Some children may benefit from a "preteaching" session during which you pass around various objects while discussing how the items feel.

2. FOLLOW THE DIRECTIONS

Objective

Child will use eye contact in communication.

Materials

- ☐ popsicle sticks
- ☐ markers
- ☐ opaque cup
- ☐ list of directions
- ☐ objects listed in directions
- ☐ large piece of paper (optional)
- ☐ glue (optional)

Procedure

Prior to the session, mark each child's name on the end of a popsicle stick. Place the sticks in a cup with the names pointed down so they are hidden. Make a list of simple directions you can give the children to follow and gather the necessary objects. Examples of directions might be: "Stand up, hop to the bucket, bring me the red ball." "Crawl to the door and bring me the circle" or "Stand up, walk to the sink, and bring me a paper towel."

Arrange the objects in the appropriate places around the room. Explain to the children that they will each get a turn to follow some directions, but they must look you in the eye as you tell them the directions. Demonstrate eye contact with the children to be sure they understand, explaining that they won't get to hear all the directions if they don't look at you.

Choose a popsicle stick and call out the child's name. Look at the child, cueing for eye contact, if needed. Tell the child a set of

directions, then watch as the directions are performed. Encourage cheering and clapping for each child after completion of
directions.

> *Variation:* After all children have had their turn, get a large
> piece of paper and draw a rough sketch of the room. Have
> each child look at you while naming the object he or she
> found on his or her turn. Let each child glue the object he
> or she found to the paper, showing where it was found in
> the room.

3. GUESS WHO?

Objective

Child will use eye contact in communication.

Materials

- ☐ stickers
- ☐ sticker chart

Procedure

Have the children sit in a circle on the floor. Explain that this is a guessing game. Tell them that you will describe someone in the group, and the others must guess who you are describing. However, you can only describe someone who is looking at you. For example, say "Guess who has a . . . pause, and see who is looking at you, then add a description of that child: ". . . red shirt." Let the children guess who it is, and explain that you chose that child because he or she was looking at you. After a child is "guessed," allow him or her to place a sticker on the sticker chart. Prompt eye contact for those not engaging in eye contact, demonstrating as needed, so that all children get a chance to play.

4. DICE TALK

Objective

Child will use eye contact in communication.

Materials

- ☐ a small-sized box
- ☐ plain paper to cover box
- ☐ marker
- ☐ tape

Procedure

Find a small box that can be covered with paper and used as a dice for this communication game. Use a size that is easy and fun for little hands to toss. Wrap the box in plain paper. On the faces of the dice, write questions or statements to elicit answers from the children. For example, on the six faces of the dice, you could write:

Name an animal that lives in the zoo.

Tell me a food you like to eat.

What animal lives on a farm?

What is something you like to drink?

Tell me an animal that lives on a farm.

Name a toy you like to play with.

Explain to the children that they each will get a turn to toss the dice, and they get to answer the question that lands on top. Tell them that they will answer to you, and they must look in your eyes as they talk to you. Explain that looking at people as they talk to them is a good thing we all need to practice.

Demonstrate tossing the dice and read them the question that lands on top. Show them how you answer the question while demonstrating eye-contact with each child.

Begin with a child's turn, and let him or her toss the dice. Read the child the question, and allow time for an answer. Exclaim over and praise their answers. If they do not use eye-contact while answering, tell them, "What a great answer! Now look at me while you tell me that again." If additional assistance is needed to establish eye contact, model the game for them and have them imitate you. Some children may benefit from having a wall poster to look at depicting possible answers (farm animals, zoo animals, foods, toys, and drinks).

5. CLOWN DAY

Objective

Child will use eye contact in communication.

Materials

☐ face paint or makeup

☐ clothing or costumes

☐ stuffed animals or puppets

☐ boxes painted like circus train cars

☐ pictures of clowns

☐ mirror

☐ camera

Procedure

The teacher may dress up like a clown with face make-up. Have each child sit across from the teacher, making eye contact while their face is painted. Allow the child to choose colors, designs, and extent of painting, always encouraging eye contact when making choices. Allow each child to dress like a clown by asking for clothing with eye contact.

Use the stuffed animals or puppets to act as the circus animals. Place the animals in the train and have a circus train move through "town." Take pictures of each child and the group. Encourage the children to look at the camera for the pictures.

6. DON'T DO THAT!

Objective

Child will use eye contact in communication.

Materials

☐ noncarbonated drink mix

☐ sugar or sweetener as per directions on mix

☐ water as per directions on mix

☐ a pitcher, ice

☐ sand

☐ rocks

☐ brown liquid (weak tea)

Procedure

Tell the children that you are going to make something to drink and that you need their help. Give each child an ingredient. Read the recipe for making the drink, including only the appropriate ingredients. Begin to make the drink and ask the children if sand should go into the pitcher. Encourage eye contact as each item is requested. Encourage eye contact as ingredients are rejected.

> *Variation:* Try other simple recipes with other wrong ingredients.

7. WOULD YOU EAT THAT?

Objective

Child will use eye contact in communication.

Materials

- ☐ *Gregory the Terrible Eater* (by M. Sharmat [1980] Scholastic, Inc., New York)
- ☐ 4 ounces or cream cheese
- ☐ ⅓ cup of sour cream
- ☐ 2 tablespoons tomato juice
- ☐ 1 tablespoon dry Italian or Ranch salad dressing mix
- ☐ assorted raw vegetables
- ☐ mixing bowl
- ☐ large spoon
- ☐ measuring cups
- ☐ spoons

Procedure

Read the book with the children. It is a story about a goat that prefers vegetables, fruit, eggs, and fish. His parents want him to eat boxes, shoes, pants, and tin cans. Ask the children, "Do you eat _____?" Encourage eye contact as they respond with yes or no. Give each child an ingredient, and assign a child to be the cook who directs the preparation. Encourage eye contact as each item is requested.

Variation: Try other similar books and other recipes.

8. CHILDREN, BE GOOD!

Objective

Child will use eye contact in communication.

Materials

- ☐ doll
- ☐ pretend food
- ☐ other props that might be helpful

Procedure

Discuss rules with children and why rules are important. Ask them what rules they have at home (or ask the parents ahead of time). Role-play with the children and doll. You will be the child and the children will be the parents. Pretend to break rules such as arguing with siblings (doll), making a mess. The children are to be encouraged to pretend to be the parent and to tell the child "no" with appropriate eye contact.

9. BABY ANIMALS STORY

Objective

Child will use eye contact in communication.

Materials

☐ book depicting baby animals with their mothers

Procedure

Read the book to the children. Ask the children if the adult animal is the baby's mother. Encourage appropriate eye contact when they respond to the question.

Variation: Use pictures of the children's parents and siblings as stimuli.

10. BUNDLE UP

Objective

Child will use eye contact in communication.

Materials

- ☐ coats,
- ☐ gloves,
- ☐ hats,
- ☐ scarves, and
- ☐ boots belonging to the children

Procedure

Before going outside to play or to get on the bus to go home, gather all of the children's outer wear in to a pile. Hold up one item at a time and ask "Whose _____ is this?" Encourage eye contact as each item is presented.

> *Hint:* Make sure you know which items belong to each child before placing them in the pile.

Turn Taking

1. SINGING SIMPLE SONGS

Objective

Child will use turn taking in a group activity.

Materials

☐ a wall chart that has a picture to associate with each song

Procedure

Sit in a circle on the floor. Lead the children in songs that they know well and have actions to keep their little hands busy while singing. If you are not familiar with actions for the song, make up appropriate actions to demonstrate as you sing (they will enjoy copying you). Movements throughout the song facilitate the children staying seated in their spots on the floor, and it also gives children who don't sing a way to remain involved in the activity.

As you begin each new song, point to the picture on the wall associated with it.

After you have sung the same songs over several days and the children are familiar with them, allow the children to take turns choosing which song to sing next by pointing to the picture on the wall chart.

> *Hint:* Keep the songs and actions very simple and easily learned.

Examples of Songs

"Row, Row, Row Your Boat" (move your arms in rowing motion as you sing) When children become more familiar with this activity, include variations of songs such as "fast" or "slow".

"If You're Happy and You Know It" (clap your hands, stomp your feet, shout hooray)

"Itsy, Bitsy Spider" (finger play spider climbing, being washed out, etc.)

"Are You Sleeping, Brother John?" (Eyes closed, folded hands at side of head, then shake hands as if ringing bell at end)

"Heads, Shoulders, Knees and Toes" Use variations such as fast/slow, loud/soft

"There Is Thunder" (tune: "Where is Thumpkin?")

"There is thunder" (pound hands on floor)

"There is thunder

Hear it roar

Hear it roar

Pitter patter raindrops" (snap fingers)

"Pitter patter raindrops

I'm all wet!" (shake wet hands)

"I'm all wet!"

"Five Little Monkeys" (finger play)

"Five little monkeys swinging in the tree" (swing 5 fingers in air)

"Teasing Mr. Alligator, 'Ya can't catch me, no you can't catch me!'

"Along came Mr. Alligator, quiet as can be" (other hand sneaks up quietly on monkeys)

"Snaps that monkey right out of the tree!"

Repeat with 4 little monkeys, then 3, and so on.

"Grandma's Spectacles" (finger play)

"Here are grandma's spectacles" (fingers around eyes like glasses)

"Here is grandma's hat" (hands on head like hat)

"Here's the way she folds her hands

And puts them in her lap.

Here are Grandpa's spectacles" (fingers around eyes)

"Here is Grandpa's hat" (hands on head)

"Here's the way he folds his arms

And sits like that."

Hint: Contrast her soft voice and his loud voice.

---

2. FARM SONG AND PLAY

Objective

Child will use turn taking in a group activity.

Materials

☐ farm set with a variety of miniature farm animals

Procedure

Hide the animals in a bag. Show the children the empty barn and tell them they will use a song to take turns finding all the animals that go into the barn.

Sit in a circle on the floor and tell the children they get to sing "Old MacDonald Had a Farm" with each child adding an animal that belongs on the farm. It may be helpful to have a chart on the wall depicting the farm animals you have in the bag in case some children have trouble independently thinking of appropriate animals.

Begin the song, pausing when you come to the first, ". . . and on his farm he had a . . ." Ask the first child to name an animal that might be on the farm, then produce that animal from the bag, and allow that child to place the animal in the barn. Continue with the song, making the noises that each animal makes. Continue until each child has had a turn naming an animal. At the conclusion of the song, allow the children to engage in playing farm, moderating their actions as needed.

3. ANIMAL IMITATION

Objective

Child will use turn taking in a group activity.

Materials

- ☐ a variety of small plastic animals
- ☐ a bag to hide the animals in

Procedure

In this game, the children take turns blindly choosing an animal from the bag. At each turn, the child tells the sound the animal makes, and all the others in the group imitate that sound. Next, the child shows how that animal moves, and the whole group imitates the animal moving around the room.

> *Hint:* It helps to have a table or other large designated object that the group travels around before ending up back at the seating area. Also, be sure to include a wide variety of animals with differing methods of movement (crawling, hopping, slithering, etc.).

4. STONE SOUP

Objective

Child will use turn taking in a group activity.

Materials

- ☐ storybook with the story of "Stone Soup"
- ☐ large pot with water
- ☐ vegetables listed in the story
- ☐ a stone for each child
- ☐ long-handled spoons or sticks for stirring
- ☐ a premade pot of Stone Soup ready to eat.

Procedure

Make the pot of soup prior to the activity and have it heated and ready to eat. Have another set of vegetables available that the children will use to add to the "pretend" soup they make during the reading of the story. Show the children the large pot with water, and tell them they will get to take turns helping making a type of soup the story will tell them about. Distribute a stone and vegetables to the children. Tell them they are in charge of adding the vegetables to the soup when the story tells them to. Read the story, cueing each child to add his or her vegetables at the appropriate time. At the conclusion, allow the children to stir the pretend soup with the long spoons, while describing how long the soup would have to cook to soften the vegetables before the soup could be eaten. Tell them that you will share the Stone Soup you made the day before so they can see how good it tastes. All sit down and enjoy Stone Soup!

5. PASS THE MUSIC

Objective

Child will use turn taking in a group activity.

Materials

☐ musical instruments such as a xylophone and a drum; a maraca for each child

Procedure

Sit in a circle on the floor. Show the children the xylophone and play a short tune for them. Ask who else would like a turn and see all the hands raise. Tell the children they all will have a chance to play, but they will have to take turns. Begin with one child, allowing him or her to play the xylophone before passing it to the next child. (Allow them to play freestyle without regard to their musical skill.) Go around the entire circle, then bring out the drum and do the same. Discuss the difference in sound between the two instruments. At the conclusion of the activity, play a song from tape or CD, distribute a maraca to each child, and allow them to play along until the song concludes.

6. HOT POTATO BALL

Objective

Child will use turn taking in a group activity.

Materials

☐ Playground ball

Procedure

Have the group sit in a large circle on the floor. Demonstrate rolling the ball across the circle to a child on the other side. Tell the children they are to pretend that the ball is very hot, so they must roll the ball quickly to another child every time it comes to them.

7. CLIMB THE MOUNTAIN

Objective

Child will use turn taking in a group activity.

Materials

☐ a low bench

☐ a large tumbling mat

Procedure

Drape the mat over the bench to form an incline that can be climbed by the children. Have the children line up and take turns "climbing the mountain." Demonstrate going to the back of the line after completing the climb, explaining that they will get more turns after all the children in front of them have climbed.

Variation: When caterpillars are available outdoors, bring some in and allow the children to observe them crawling. Tell the children to pretend they are caterpillars crawling over the mountain.

---

8. BOWLING

Objective

Child will use turn taking in a group activity.

Materials

☐ plastic bowling pins and ball

☐ masking tape

Procedure

Set up the pins, placing a piece of tape on the floor to mark where the children should stand when throwing the ball. Arrange the children in a line behind the masking tape. Explain that each child will get a turn when he or she steps up to the line. Show the children how to go to the back of the line after their turn. If there are so many children that the wait in line is quite long, have two bowling sets to increase the children's turn taking and lessen the demand on their patience.

9. BOARD GAMES

Objective

Child will use turn taking in a group activity.

Materials

☐ simple board games

Procedure

Read the rules for the game to the children. Reiterate the need for patience as each child waits for his or her turn. Reward patience with praise, if possible, or with a token, if necessary.

10. OBSTACLE COURSE

Objective

Child will use turn taking in a group activity.

Materials

- ☐ carpet squares or tumbling mats
- ☐ small slide
- ☐ indoor gym set
- ☐ rocking chair
- ☐ objects hanging from the ceiling just out of reach
- ☐ beanbag chair, table, or any other furniture items

Procedure

Create an obstacle course with the materials mentioned above. Instruct the children that they are to go through the course one at a time. Have the children climb under the table, hop on the squares, rock in the chair, and so forth. Encourage the children to label the actions to build verb vocabulary as they move through the course. Remind the other children to wait for their turn.

Pretend Play

1. FAMILY FUN

Objective

Child will participate in pretend play with the group.

Materials

- ☐ oversize dress up clothes
- ☐ dolls
- ☐ stuffed animals
- ☐ kitchen set
- ☐ house play set
- ☐ other household items

Procedures

Assist the children in choosing a family member to portray while pretending. Facilitate each child's attempts to pretend. Model the actions and language appropriate for each family member.

2. ZOOKEEPER

Objective

Child will participate in pretend play with the group.

Materials

- ☐ zoo animal puppets
- ☐ pith helmets
- ☐ cardboard fencing
- ☐ plastic food items

Procedures

Make simple picket fences from cardboard. Let the children paint the fencing. Once dry, facilitate each child's choices to be animals or zookeepers. The zookeepers need to get the animals in their cages and feed them. Encourage the children to name the animals as they fence them in and feed them. Encourage the animals to make animal appropriate noises.

3. FARMER IN THE DELL

Objective

Child will participate in pretend play with the group.

Materials

- ☐ farmer's hat
- ☐ apron
- ☐ baby's hat
- ☐ dog ears
- ☐ cat ears
- ☐ mouse nose and whiskers
- ☐ cheese

Procedure

Help each child assume a role and lead them through the song, "Farmer in the Dell." Change roles and repeat several times.

"Farmer in the Dell"

"The farmer in the dell, the farmer in the dell, hi ho the derry-o, the farmer in the dell.

The farmer takes a wife . . .

The wife takes a child . . .

The child takes a dog . . .

The dog takes a cat . . .

The cat takes a mouse . . .

The mouse takes the cheese . . .

The cheese stands alone . . ."

4. I AM A PET . . . WHO AM I?

Objective

Child will participate in pretend play with the group.

Materials

☐ pictures of typical pets

Procedure

Let each child pick a picture and pretend to be the animal while the teacher "guesses" what the child is. Make several wrong guesses to facilitate continued pretend play. Include other children in the guessing, if appropriate.

Hint: The teacher may have to demonstrate how to pretend to be different animals.

5. BABY BATH AND BEDTIME

Objective

Child will participate in pretend play with the group.

Materials

- ☐ dolls
- ☐ bottles
- ☐ baby clothes
- ☐ small tubs with water
- ☐ towels

Procedure

Explain that it is bath time and the babies need their baths. Give each child a doll, tub, towels, bottles, and so forth. Model how to give the baby a bath, dry the baby, dress the baby, and feed the baby. Facilitate each child as he or she pretends to care for the baby.

6. WHAT'S FOR DINNER?

Objective

Child will participate in pretend play with the group.

Materials

- ☐ toy stove
- ☐ pots and pans
- ☐ dishes
- ☐ food items
- ☐ bowls
- ☐ spoons
- ☐ forks
- ☐ cooking utensils

Procedure

Help the children decide what to have for dinner. Have each child choose what he or she wants to "cook" and help the child pretend to prepare that item and then serve it. One child can be assigned to set the table for dinner.

7. SHOPPING DAY

Objective

Child will participate in pretend play with the group.

Materials

- ☐ pretend food/clothes/toys
- ☐ child-sized grocery carts
- ☐ list of items to buy
- ☐ cash register
- ☐ play money

Procedure

Designate one child as the cashier. Have the other children make lists of what they need to buy. Then have each child shop, getting only items on his or her list. Once all of the items are chosen, have the child pay the cashier.

> *Hint:* Do not focus on the value of items. Let the child give whatever money he or she chooses to the cashier. Instead of writing the names of items, pictures of items can be pasted to the list prior to shopping.

8. CAR WASH

Objective

Child will participate in pretend play with the group.

Materials

- ☐ toy cars
- ☐ small washtubs
- ☐ towels

Procedure

Explain that the cars are dirty and need to be washed. Let each child wash and dry several cars before parking them. If possible, let the children get the cars dirty by driving them through potting soil or sand that is slightly damp.

9. LET'S HAVE A CIRCUS PARADE!

Objective

Child will participate in pretend play with the group.

Materials

- ☐ animal puppets
- ☐ top hat
- ☐ tutus
- ☐ clown wigs
- ☐ other costumes

Procedure

Allow each child to choose who or what he or she wants to be in the circus. The ring master wears the top hat and leads the parade. Assist the animals in making appropriate animals sounds. Facilitate walking in a line around the room. If possible, move outside the room. Let the children change roles and have another parade.

10. MUSIC TIME

Objective

Child will participate in pretend play with the group.

Materials

☐ child-sized musical instruments (drum, tambourine, triangle, bell, horns, maracas, xylophone)

Procedure

Demonstrate how to play each instrument. Give each child a choice between two instruments. Make sure you have at least one extra instrument so that each child gets a choice.

Count to three and say "Go!" Have the children walk in a circle, playing until the teacher says "Stop!" Everyone stops walking and playing until the teacher says "go!" again. Repeat several times. Count to three but pause before saying "go!" to see if any of the children will direct the group to go.

CHAPTER 3

Activities for Children Six to Nine Years of Age

Cooperative Skills

1. GUESS THAT SOUND

Objective

Child will use cooperative skills in a group activity.

Materials

- ☐ a variety of objects that make recognizable noises, such as a xylophone, a cup of water being poured, a bell, a telephone, a clock ticking, etc.
- ☐ a screen to hide the noisemakers
- ☐ stickers
- ☐ a sticker chart
- ☐ a "noisy" snack such as potato chips, carrots, celery, popcorn, etc.

Procedure

Inform the children that they will hear noises, and they must act as a team to guess the objects making the noise. Explain that it will help to talk things over with each other, getting ideas about what the sound might be. Each time the group correctly guesses an item, a sticker will be added to the sticker chart. When the chart is full, treat everyone to a noisy snack!

> *Variations:* Allow the child who guessed correctly to place the sticker on the board; designate a different child as spokesperson for the group, instructing the nonspokespersons to tell the spokesperson their guess for revealing aloud; play a tape of simple recognizable noises.

2. FEELIE FINGERS

Objective

Child will use cooperative skills in a group activity.

Materials

- ☐ one large piece of butcher paper
- ☐ marker
- ☐ safety scissors
- ☐ glue
- ☐ plastic
- ☐ sandpaper
- ☐ cotton
- ☐ various fabrics with textures

Procedure

Draw a large hand on the butcher paper. Give each child scissors and various textured fabrics. Assign each child a finger to be in charge of, meaning that each finger should have one texture. Each child is encouraged to cut the materials into pieces. The child in charge of the thumb, for example, will direct the others to put the corduroy on the thumb. The teacher should facilitate gluing of the materials to each finger.

3. FEELIE FLOWER

Objective

Child will use cooperative skills in a group activity.

Materials

- ☐ large piece of butcher paper
- ☐ various fabrics with different textures (velvet, dotted swiss, corduroy, burlap, satin)
- ☐ safety scissors
- ☐ glue sticks (one or two to encourage sharing)

Procedure

Draw a large daisy-type flower on the butcher paper. Give each child pieces of each fabric. Allow the children to determine how the fabrics will be placed on the flower. Each petal could be a collage of fabrics or each could be made from one fabric only. A stem and leaves can be added and the same decisions can be made by the children. Encourage the children to work together to complete the flower and to share the glue sticks.

4. NO-COOK FUDGE

Objective

Child will use cooperative skills in a group activity.

Materials

- ☐ 1 cup powdered sugar
- ☐ 2 tablespoons cocoa
- ☐ ⅛ cup peanut butter
- ☐ 1 tablespoon milk
- ☐ mixing bowl
- ☐ wooden spoon
- ☐ measuring spoons and cups

Procedure

Assign each child one ingredient for the fudge. Facilitate each child's measurement and addition of ingredients. Allow each child an opportunity to stir the mixture. Let each child roll spoonfuls into balls and refrigerate any leftovers.

> *Variations:* Crunchy peanut butter adds a different texture. Children can press fudge into candy molds to make different shapes. Fudge can be pressed flat and cut with cookie cutters. The molds and cutters can be related to a theme (animals, flowers, transportation, etc.).

5. LEAF PRINTS

Objective

Child will use cooperative skills in a group activity.

Materials

- ☐ leaves of different shapes
- ☐ newspaper
- ☐ rolling pin
- ☐ tissue paper
- ☐ paints
- ☐ one paintbrush per color

Procedure

Give each child several pieces of newspaper. Place paints, brushes, and leaves where each child can reach them. Instruct the children to pick a leaf and a paint color. Demonstrate how to paint the leaf and place it paint side up on the newspaper. Cover the leaf with the tissue paper and roll with the rolling pin. Encourage the children to share the paint colors and rolling pin. Consider letting each child be in charge of an item so they have to work together to complete the activity.

6. HOUSE COLLAGE

Objective

Child will use cooperative skills in a group activity.

Materials

- ☐ one large piece of butcher paper with a simple house drawn on it with a living room, kitchen, bathroom and bedroom
- ☐ magazine pictures of furniture, appliances, plumbing fixtures, etc.
- ☐ one or two pairs of safety scissors
- ☐ one or two glue sticks

Procedure

Allow the group to determine which room is which and label each. Facilitate the discussion of furnishings, appliances, and so forth for each room. Consider placing one child in charge of each room to direct the furnishing of each room. Encourage sharing of the scissors and glue sticks.

7. MUSICAL CHAIRS

Objective

Child will use cooperative skills in a group activity.

Materials

☐ chairs arranged in a circle with spaces between

☐ music CDs or tapes

☐ CD or tape player

Procedure

Offer the children the opportunity to be the "teacher" and control the music. If no one chooses this role, the teacher should assume the role. Explain the rules of the game, perhaps writing them down, and explaining that whoever does not get a chair can help with the music. Remind the children to remember that, "Sometimes I win, sometimes I lose. It is just fun to play the game." Play until one child is left, and then repeat.

8. SPONGE PAINTING AN OCEAN

Objective

Child will use cooperative skills in a group activity.

Materials

- ☐ sponges cut into fish, coral, and seaweed shapes
- ☐ tempera paints in shallow containers
- ☐ paper towels
- ☐ large piece of butcher paper painted blue and allowed to dry

Procedure

Read a book or look at pictures depicting the ocean. Place a paper towel in each shallow container and pour in a small amount of tempera paint to make a paint pad. Let the children dip the various sponges in the paints and press them onto the butcher paper.

> *Hint:* Foam meat trays, cleaned with bleach solution, work well as paint trays. Precut sponges may be available at craft stores. Small wooden beads can be hot-glued to the sponges to act a handles. Neon-colored paints work well on the blue background.

9. SCARECROW FOR THE FALL

Objective

Child will use cooperative skills in a group activity.

Materials

- ☐ pair of pants
- ☐ long-sleeved T-shirt
- ☐ hat
- ☐ gloves
- ☐ baby-sized pillowcase
- ☐ rubber bands
- ☐ straw, marker
- ☐ shower curtain liner or drop cloth if done inside

Procedures

Place rubber bands around the bottom of the pant legs and around the shirt neck and cuffs. Help the children work together to stuff the pants, shirt, pillowcase, and gloves. Pull a few pieces of straw through the pant legs for feet. Use another rubber band to attach the gloves to the sleeves. Following directions from the children, draw a face on the pillowcase and place it on the shirt neck using rubber bands. Place the hat on the head. Put the scarecrow in a chair.

> *Hint:* Have a needle and strong thread handy to affix the head to the shirt and hat to the head, if necessary. Place the scarecrow outside in a garden space if possible.

10. TRAIL MIX

Objective

Child will use cooperative skills in a group activity.

Materials

- ☐ bowls or disposable, containers with lids
- ☐ trail mix ingredients such as cereal bits, nuts, raisins, chocolate/peanut butter/butterscotch bits, dried fruit bits, coconut
- ☐ coffee scoops
- ☐ measuring cups or spoons
- ☐ marker

Procedure

Give each child a bowl. Place food items into bowls with scoops, cups, or spoons. Let each child be in charge of a food item to encourage interaction. Allow each child to make his or her own version of trail mix by asking for each ingredient. Encourage the children to try any food they are not sure about. Have the snack! Place leftovers in zipper-style bags if bowls were used or place the lids on containers, and help the children label the containers with their names.

Eye-Contact

1. HOW DO YOU DO?

Objective

Child will use eye contact while speaking and listening.

Materials

None

Procedure

Have the group sit on the floor in a circle. The leader gets up, walks around the outside of the circle to a target person, then reaches out to shake hands with target person. The target person stands to face the leader. While shaking hands and looking into the eyes of target person, leader says, "How do you do, how do you do, how do you do." The target person replies, while looking into eyes of leader, "I'm fine, I'm fine, I'm fine." The two people then walk quickly in opposite directions to the space left empty by the target person; the first one there sits down, and other person continues game as leader.

Group members may need occasional reminders to keep using eye contact as the game continues. Encourage leaders to pick children who have not yet been chosen.

2. EYE TO EYE, PEOPLE TO PEOPLE

Objective

Child will use eye contact while speaking and listening.

Materials

None

Procedure

Tell students that this game will help them practice the important communication skill of eye contact. Pair each student with a partner, explaining that they will be switching partners throughout the game. Students stand in a circle, next to their partners. The leader stands in the middle.

The leader calls out body parts, such as "Hand to hand," "Back to back," "Elbow to knee," and so on, and the partners must put together the two body parts named. After calling out a few different body parts, leader calls out, "Eye to eye," during which partners must look into each other's eyes. Leader must count 1, 1,000; 2, 1,000; 3, 1,000, 4, 1,000; 5, 1,000 so that eye contact lasts for 5 seconds. Then leader calls, "People to people!" at which time group members scramble to find a new partner. The last one to find a partner is the new leader.

3. MIRROR GAME

Objective

Child will use eye contact while speaking and listening.

Materials

☐ timer

Procedure

Pair each student with a partner. Have partners sit in chairs facing each other. Designate one partner in each pair as the leader for the first round. Their partners are thus the "mirrors" for the first round. Explain that the leader and partner must look each other in the eye for one minute. During this time, the leader moves his or her head and face in various ways; the partner mimics all movements, making it appear as if the leader is looking into a mirror.

Demonstrate with a partner to show students the mirror effect; use slow, exaggerated head and facial movements such as raising the eyebrows, smiling, opening the mouth, tilting the head side to side, blinking the eyes, grimacing, closing one eye at a time, and so forth. Emphasize that students must continue looking into each other's eyes for the entire minute of each round.

Set the timer for one minute. At the end of each round, have students switch roles so each child has a chance to play the leader and the mirror. After the second round, students may switch partners to begin a new experience of leader and mirror.

4. WHOSE FOOTPRINTS?

Objective

Child will use eye contact while speaking and listening.

Materials

- ☐ large tub with about 2 inches of water in it
- ☐ 2 large sheets of butcher paper (one about 6 feet long)
- ☐ tempera paints
- ☐ small paint rollers

Procedure

Tell the children they are going to make their own footprints. Tell them that, to get their feet painted, they have to look at the teacher. The teacher will say, "Whose footprints?" to each child. When the child looks at the teacher, his or her feet will get painted. Then the child will walk down the 6-foot-long paper making prints. The child will then step into the tub at the end of the print paper and wash his or her feet. The child may go through again once everyone has had a turn.

5. HOW DO I MOVE?

Objective

Child will use eye contact while speaking and listening.

Materials

☐ list of animals or pictures of animals

Procedure

Discuss the ways that different animals move. Have the children act out different animal movements. Once the children have done this, tell them that they are to choose an animal from pictures or a list and then move like that animal. The other children will raise their hands to guess the animal, and the actor will call on the children to guess. Emphasize that the actor and the guesser need to look at each other when choosing and guessing.

6. LOOK WHAT I CAN DO!

Objective

Child will use eye contact while speaking and listening.

Materials

☐ any book depicting children doing various actions (jumping, running, hopping, sliding, swinging, clapping, pointing, reading, etc.)

Procedure

Read the book to the children. Reread the book and tell the children that when you look at them, they get to do the action. Have the child label the action, if possible. Wait until the child looks at the teacher before giving him or her the action to portray.

7. FAVORITE ANIMALS

Objective

Child will use eye contact while speaking and listening.

Materials

- ☐ each child brings a favorite stuffed animal from home
- ☐ construction paper cutouts of animal bodies, heads, and paws
- ☐ two glue sticks
- ☐ two markers
- ☐ buttons
- ☐ sheets of construction paper

Procedure

Discuss each cutout part and give all the bodies to one child, the heads to another, and so on. Give each child a sheet of paper and let the children ask each other for the various parts they need. Tell the children they have to look at the person they are asking. If the child does not speak, eye contact will suffice to get the various parts needed. Limit the glue sticks and markers available to facilitate requesting among the children.

8. A BOOK ABOUT ME

Objective

Child will use eye contact while speaking and listening.

Materials

☐ any book focusing on body parts

Procedure

Read the book and have the children point to their body parts when they are named in the book. Reread the book and tell the children that when the teacher looks at them, they are to point to the part that matches the book. Remind them to look at the teacher so they will know when it is their turn.

9. RED LIGHT, GREEN LIGHT

Objective

Child will use eye contact while speaking and listening.

Materials

None

Procedure

Tell the children that they can jump or hop or walk when the teacher holds up a "Green Light," but they must stop when the teacher holds up, "Red Light." Tell them they have to look at the teacher to know when they can move. The children can then take turns being the teacher.

10. FOLLOW THE LEADER

Objective

Child will use eye contact while speaking and listening.

Materials

None

Procedure

Have the children line up side-by-side facing the teacher. Tell the children to do what the teacher does. Mix more visible, gross motor movements with more subtle, fine motor movements such as facial expressions. Remind the children that they have to look at the teacher to know what to do. Let each child take a turn as the teacher.

Facial Expressions

1. READ MY FACE

Objective

Child will use facial expressions to convey feelings.

Materials

None

Procedure

The teacher tells a story involving people who are experiencing many different emotions. At key points in the story where the characters experience emotions, the teacher pauses to dramatize the characters' facial expressions. Students take part by identifying and imitating facial expressions. At the end of the story, students take turns re-enacting the characters' facial expressions as the teacher repeats the story.

Stories may be preplanned or impromptu. A sample story follows:

"At the first Thanksgiving, a little Pilgrim girl was sent out to gather berries to make pies for the big feast. She skipped happily through the forest looking for ripe, plump berries." (Pause to dramatize skipping with happy facial expression, have students imitate.) "She was bent low picking berries when she heard rustling in the grass behind her. Her face showed her fear as she crouched low and hid, not knowing what wild animal might be stalking her." (Pause, dramatizing crouching with fearful facial expression, ask students to imitate expression.) "When nothing pounced at her, she slowly turned to face the noise. Instead of a wild animal, she saw a little Indian child who had come to share Thanksgiving with the Pilgrims. She had never met a real Indian before, and the girl shrieked in surprise." (Pause, dramatize surprised face, have students imitate.) "The little Indian child saw the bucket and started picking berries to help the girl. When the bucket was full, the girl and the Indian walked to the Thanksgiving feast hand in hand, each happy to have made a new friend." (Pause to dramatize happy face, have students imitate.)

2. PASS THAT FACE

Objective

Child will use facial expressions to convey feelings.

Materials

☐ slips of paper

☐ pen

☐ small bowl

Procedure

On the slips of paper, write various emotions that are often conveyed via facial expressions. Examples: happy, sad, mad, surprised, frustrated, confused. Put the slips of paper into a small bowl.

Have the children sit in a circle on the floor. Explain that, one at a time, they will take turns drawing a slip of paper and reading the emotion listed on it. They are then to turn to the person on their left, state the feeling aloud, and use their faces to show that feeling. That person then turns to the person on his or her left, states the feeling, and makes a face to match the feeling. The next person then does the same to the person on his or her left, until the face has been passed around the entire circle.

3. EXPRESSION CHARADES

Objective

Child will use facial expressions to convey feelings.

Materials

- ☐ slips of paper
- ☐ pen
- ☐ bowl to hold slips of paper

Procedure

This adaptation of the game of charades allows students to practice using and reading communicative facial expressions. Write the expressions you wish students to practice on small slips of paper. Suggestions include happy, angry, confused, frustrated, surprised, and mischievous. Place the slips in a small bowl. Have the children sit in a circle. Instruct them that each will get a turn to choose a slip of paper from the bowl, and they should not show or tell anyone what it says. The child must then use his or her face to show the feeling listed on the paper, while the other students try to guess the feeling. Allow guessing to continue as long as you feel appropriate for each child and the group. Give hints if a turn takes too long or if a child encounters difficulty.

4. EXPRESS YOURSELF

Objective

Child will use facial expressions to convey feelings.

Materials

- ☐ different colors of construction paper
- ☐ marker or pen
- ☐ music tape
- ☐ tape player

Procedure

On the construction paper, write brief descriptions of situations that would evoke various emotions in a child. Examples:

"You are in line to buy lunch at school and you realize you forgot your lunch money."

"You pull out your winter coat on the first day of cold weather, reach into the pocket and find a $20 bill."

"You are trying to glue together a model car but it keeps falling apart."

Include as many colors of paper, and therefore that many descriptive situations, as you have children. Place the pieces of construction paper face down in circle, about one footstep apart. Tell the children that you will play music and they are to walk around the circle stepping on the construction papers until the music stops. When the music stops, call out a color. Whoever is standing on that color reads the scenario aloud. The child is then instructed to make a facial expression to depict the emotion he or she would feel if the situation happened to them. Instruct all of the children in the group to then imitate that facial expression.

5. TEDDY BEAR SONG

Objective

Child will use facial expressions to convey feelings.

Materials

None

Procedure

Demonstrate the Teddy Bear chant. Insert different facial movements and expressions in the activity.

Teddy Bear Chant

Teddy Bear, Teddy Bear make a big smile.

Teddy Bear, Teddy Bear stick out your tongue.

(and so on)

6. TRACK MEET

Objective

Child will use facial expressions to convey feelings.

Materials

- ☐ balloons
- ☐ drinking straws
- ☐ long stick
- ☐ paper plates
- ☐ feathers
- ☐ medals

Procedure

Plan a track meet using various objects for the categories suggested below.

Shot put with water balloons

Javelin throw using straws

Discus throw using paper plates

Standing broad grins (measure smiles)

Feather-blow relay

Limbo contest under the long stick

Hopping or standing on one foot

Name and describe each activity as it is being completed. Talk about being happy when you win and how it is okay if you do not win. "Sometimes we win, sometimes we lose. It is just fun to play the game."

7. HOW DO I FEEL?

Objective

Child will use facial expressions to convey feelings.

Materials

- ☐ two pairs of safety scissors
- ☐ paper plates
- ☐ two sets of crayons
- ☐ hole punch
- ☐ string

Procedure

Model various facial expressions. Have the children guess what emotion is being modeled. Discuss how the children knew what emotion it was by looking at the expression on your face. Have the children try to make several facial expressions. Have the children draw happy, sad, and mad faces on the paper plates. Encourage sharing of the scissors and crayons. Punch holes in the top of the plates, cut a length of string to make a loose necklace, and attach it to the plate. Hang the plate faces around the children's necks and let them take turns showing their happy faces, sad faces, and so forth.

8. IF YOU ARE HAPPY AND YOU KNOW IT!

Objective

Child will use facial expressions to convey feelings.

Materials

None

Procedure

Sing the song and insert facial expressions and head movements in each verse.

Make a smile.

Stick out your tongue.

Nod your head.

Close your eyes.

Have the children act out each expression or movement. Remind the children to look at the teacher so they will know what to do. Have the children label each expression or movement, if possible.

9. CATS ON THE FENCE

Objective

Child will use facial expressions to convey feelings.

Materials

None

Procedure

Teach the song to the children.

"When everyone is fast asleep,"

(Clasp hands, put them up to cheek and tilt head and smile)

"My cat goes out to play.

He leaps up on the tall, high fence"

(Jump in place, look surprised)

"And walks along the way."

(Walk in place)

"First one foot and then the other"

(Lift one foot high, then the other foot high)

"Slowly walking, slowly stalking,"

(Make a serious face)

"That big white cat of mine."

(Sway body from side to side and meow after last word)

Repeat several times until the children become familiar with the words.

10. FEELINGS

Objective

Child will use facial expressions to convey feelings.

Materials

☐ any book that focuses on feelings or emotions

Procedure

Read the book and emphasize each emotion. Make the corresponding facial expression. Discuss how each emotion feels and some reasons why that emotion might occur. Have the children label different emotions and act them out.

Turn Taking

1. PUMPKIN DECORATING

Objective

Child will use turn-taking in group activity.

Materials

- ☐ one large pumpkin
- ☐ pretty fall leaves of various shapes and colors
- ☐ yarn
- ☐ markers
- ☐ construction paper
- ☐ scissors
- ☐ tape
- ☐ slips of numbered paper and a hat to draw them out of to determine turn-taking order

Procedure

Tell the group they get to decorate a pumpkin, giving it a face, hair, and ears. Instruct the children that they are free to use any of the materials, but they must take turns adding decorations to the pumpkin. Allow them a brief time to discuss possible decorating ideas; if necessary, prompt their creativity with suggestions such as, "Leaves for hair? A mouth out of yarn? Draw ears with a marker?" Draw numbers out of a hat to determine the order they go in, informing them everyone may each have as many turns as necessary to fully decorate the pumpkin.

2. FLOOR PUZZLE

Objective

Child will use turn-taking in group activity.

Materials

☐ floor puzzle with pieces large enough to be seen by all group members as they gather around puzzle on the floor. (Small puzzle pieces are not conducive to group work.)

Procedure

Distribute pieces of the puzzle randomly to each student, making sure all students end with the same number of pieces. If available, show students a picture of the completed puzzle. Explain that the group will be building the puzzle together by taking turns adding their pieces. However, students are only allowed to handle their own pieces; they are not allowed to take someone else's pieces and add to the puzzle. If they happen to see where another student's piece should go, they are allowed to make verbal suggestions and point but not touch another student's puzzle piece.

When ready to begin, ask for a volunteer to place the first piece. At this time, students will be looking at their own pieces as well as other students' pieces to spy a corner piece or some other easily recognized piece. If no one volunteers, explain that corner pieces make good beginnings and prompt the owner of a corner piece to begin. Go in circle fashion for turn-taking, but if a student is unsure of placing a piece, he or she may "pass" and allow the next person to go. In the end, all students will have had the same number of turns because they all have the same number of pieces.

3. WATCH THE LEADER

Objective

Child will use turn-taking in group activity.

Materials

None

Procedure

Have the children sit in a circle. Explain that each child will get a turn to be the "leader," and that everyone else gets to copy whatever action movement the leader makes. Explain that they must pay close attention to watching the leader, because he or she will change action movements after each little while.

Demonstrate by being the first leader. Start by performing simple actions like tapping your knees with both hands; after a few repetitions and when all children are watching you, switch to tapping your shoulders; next switch to rubbing your tummy, then patting your cheeks, pulling your ears, and so forth. Vary the complexity of the actions to be commensurate with the abilities of the group. After a few rounds, announce that your turn is finished and name the child next to you to be the leader, explaining that after his turn the child seated next to him will be the leader, and so on until everyone has taken a turn.

> *Hint:* To avoid distracting eruptions from the circle, remind the children that this is a "sit-down" game and they must stay on their spots in the circle as they game is played.

4. SANDPAPER PRINTS

Objective

Child will use turn-taking in group activity.

Materials

- ☐ crayons
- ☐ sandpaper squares
- ☐ plain white or manila paper
- ☐ iron
- ☐ newspaper section

Procedure

Allow the children to draw designs on the rough sandpaper with the crayons. Limit the number of crayons available to facilitate turn-taking. Lay a piece of the plain paper over the sandpaper and press it with the warm iron. Lift off the paper and discuss the smooth design transferred from the sandpaper to the plain paper. Remind the children to wait for their turn to have their design pressed.

Caution: The teacher must maintain strict control of the iron at all times.

5. FLY, MR. BIRD!

Objective

Child will use turn-taking in group activity.

Materials

☐ pictures of birds

☐ tongue depressors

☐ tape

Procedure

Have the students write a simple story including each of the different types of birds. The stories can be based on fact or imaginative. Make hand-held posters of the bird pictures by taping each one to a tongue depressor. Have one child narrate the story while the others assume the various roles. Each child should be reminded to wait his or her turn in the story. Each child can then take a turn as narrator.

6. SNACK WITH FEELING

Objective

Child will use turn-taking in group activity.

Materials

- ☐ paper plates
- ☐ napkins
- ☐ cups
- ☐ beverage
- ☐ various foods

    Crunchy: corn chips, celery

    Juicy: oranges, grapes, kiwi

    Soft: marshmallows, bananas, pudding

    Dry: crackers, popcorn, bread

    Hard: carrots, nuts

    Chewy: raisins, caramels, jelly beans

    Cold: ice cream

    Hot: soup

Procedure

Give each child a small amount of each food. Ask each child to take turns describing the different foods. Remind the children to listen to the others and to wait for their turn to speak.

7. SAND PICTURE AT THE BEACH

Objective

Child will use turn-taking in group activity.

Materials

- ☐ 9 × 12 white construction paper
- ☐ various other colors of construction paper
- ☐ liquid glue (slightly thinned with water)
- ☐ paint brush
- ☐ sand
- ☐ markers
- ☐ two pairs of safety scissors

Procedure

Draw a wavy horizon line across the middle of the white paper. Have the children work together to color the upper portion blue for the sky. Discuss what else is needed for the beach picture (beach umbrella, pail and shovel, palm tree, sun, beach ball, towel, etc.). Lightly paint the thinned glue across the lower portion of the white paper and allow the children to collectively sprinkle sand over the glue. Shake off the excess and then allow the children to take turns adding the assorted beach items.

8. MIXED-UP CLOTHES

Objective

Child will use turn-taking in group activity.

Materials

☐ children's clothing items brought from home

☐ paper bag or box.

Procedure

Place each child's clothing in the bag or box and naming the item and owner; each child should respond when it is his or her item of clothing. Remind the children to raise their hands and wait until they are called on to respond. The teacher can add some personal items to model appropriate responses.

9. FIRE SAFETY BOOK

Objective

Child will use turn-taking in group activity.

Materials

☐ any book about firefighters or the fire station

☐ fire helmet

☐ rubber boots

Procedures

Read the story and discuss each aspect of the firefighter's gear and/or the station. Discuss fire safety issues with the children. Let each child take a turn being the fire captain wearing the helmet and boots. Each captain can review fire safety issues to reinforce the learning objectives.

10. WIDE-EYED WORM MAGNET

Objective

Child will use turn-taking in group activity.

Materials

- ☐ wooden clothespins with spring
- ☐ small pompoms
- ☐ binder hole reinforcers
- ☐ self-adhesive magnet tape
- ☐ hot-melt glue

Procedure

Cut the magnet tape to the length of the clothespins. Let each child stick the tape to one side of the clothespin. Let the children take turns collecting different color pompoms for their worm. Let the children take turns having the teacher glue the pompoms to the clothespin. Remind the students that they must wait quietly for their turn. Give each child two binder reinforcers to be the eyes at the pincher end of the clothespin. Each child can then take a turn describing his or her worm.

Role-Play

1. POLICE VEST AND BADGE

Objective

Child will participate in role-play with the group.

Materials

- ☐ large paper bag for each child
- ☐ index card for each child
- ☐ yellow paint
- ☐ blue paint
- ☐ newspaper
- ☐ picture of police officer
- ☐ two pairs of safety scissors
- ☐ marker
- ☐ two glue sticks

Procedure

Show the group a picture of a police officer and talk about how the officer helps us. Point out the uniform and the badge. Tell the children they are going to make a police uniform to wear. Help the children cut out a neck hole and two arm holes in the bag. Help the children cut a slit up the front of the bag to make a vest. Draw star shapes on the index cards and have the children paint them yellow. Set aside to dry. Spread newspaper and have the children paint the vest blue. While the vest dries, cut out the star badge. Let the children put on the vests and affix their badges and facilitate their role-play as police officers.

> *Note:* If the vests are not dry, save them for the next time and role-play then.

2. SAFETY SALLY AND DANGEROUS DAN

Objective

Child will participate in role-play with the group.

Materials

- ☐ Safety Sally puppet
- ☐ Dangerous Dan puppet
- ☐ small toys
- ☐ carpet squares
- ☐ shoe box

Procedure

Any female and male puppets can serve as Sally and Dan. If none are available, puppets can easily be crafted from small paper bags and construction paper. Introduce Safety Sally at a time when the room needs cleaning up. Make a mini-room for Sally by placing small toys on a carpet square and have the shoe box serve as a toy chest. Let the children know that Sally is upset about the mess in her room because she is worried about someone falling and getting hurt. She is worried that toys may get broken as well. Talk about places where scattered toys are dangerous, like on the stairs, in a doorway, or in the driveway. Have Sally happily clean up the toys and put them in the toy box. Introduce Dangerous Dan who follows Sally around and makes a mess again. Let the children take turns being Dan and Sally.

3. DON'T BREAK THE LAW!

Objective

Child will participate in role-play with the group.

Materials

☐ police vests and badges from the previous activity

Procedure

Discuss laws and rules. Talk about why it is important to follow the laws and explain that rules in the classroom are like laws. Talk about what police officers do. Have the children pretend to be police officers. The teacher can be the "bad guy" and pretend to break laws. Each child can arrest the bad guy.

> *Note:* It is also not a good idea for the children to be the "bad guy" unless one is certain they understand they are only pretending.

4. WEATHER WILLIE AND WANDA

Objective

Child will participate in role-play with the group.

Materials

- ☐ flannel or magnet board of a boy and girl
- ☐ appropriate clothing for rain, winter, summer, for both figures
- ☐ frame cut of poster board to serve as TV

Procedure

One child is assigned the job of weatherperson who will report the weather so Willie and Wanda can get dressed. The weather can vary from rain to sunshine, from winter to summer. Encourage the use of descriptive language (warm, cool, hot, cold). Discuss what the boy and girl should wear depending on the weather situation. Each child can take turns being Willie or Wanda as well as the weatherperson.

5. BIG MUSCLES!

Objective

Child will participate in role-play with the group.

Materials

☐ Heavy objects and light objects

Heavy	Light
cans of soup	feathers
detergent jug	foam cups
hammer	crayon
dictionary	leaf
rock	cotton balls

Procedure

Talk about things that are heavy and light and ask the children for the meanings of each word. Children can pretend to be weightlifters and take turns lifting the objects. Each child can win a medal for his or her big muscles.

6. STOP, DROP, AND ROLL

Objective

Child will participate in role-play with the group.

Materials

None

Procedure

Discuss fire safety. Demonstrate the stop, drop, and roll method to use if a person's clothes are on fire. Have the children practice the method and describe what they are doing.

7. SAFETY AT HOME

Objective

Child will participate in role-play with the group.

Materials

☐ child-sized playhouse or small dollhouse with people

Procedure

Discuss safety rules for the home and school. The discussion can include fire safety, stranger safety, and even storm safety. Discuss what the children should do in the event of a dangerous situation. Have the children role-play what they would do if they were asleep and a fire was in their home or what to do if a stranger asks you to help him find a lost puppy. Discuss how to find an adult for help or to call 9–1–1.

> *Caution:* Some children with AS have unusual fears, and this type of role play may cause undue anxiety. Discuss with parents.

8. FIREFIGHTER FUN!

Objective

Child will participate in role-play with the group.

Materials

- ☐ helmets
- ☐ rubber boots
- ☐ raincoats

Procedure

Discuss the role of firefighters and the clothing they must wear to protect them. Discuss the various activities firefighters have to do, including driving a fire truck, using a hose, climbing ladders, rescuing people, even getting cats out of trees. Let each child dress up and pretend to be a firefighter.

9. COMMUNITY HELPERS

Objective

Child will participate in role-play with the group.

Materials

- [ ] any book about community helpers
- [ ] props for police officer, firefighter, doctor, veterinarian, nurse, librarian, teacher, and so on

Procedure

Read the book and discuss the various people who help us in our community. Discuss each helper's job the activities are associated with that job. Let each child role-play as the different community helpers using the props collected. Let the other children pretend to be the people who are helped.

10. YOU CAN BE A FARMER . . . A WORM FARMER!

Objective

Child will participate in role-play with the group.

Materials

- ☐ large jar
- ☐ black paper
- ☐ rocks
- ☐ soil
- ☐ leaves
- ☐ worms
- ☐ food for worms (used coffee grounds, lettuce, egg shells, grass clippings)

Procedure

Discuss where worms live, what they eat, and what purpose they serve in the ecology of the earth. Place all of the materials on the table and allow one child to assume to role of farmer who will instruct the farm helpers on how to build the worm farm. Place a few rocks in the bottom of the jar and add soil and dry leaves. Put several worms in the jar and note how they dive into the soil. Put in about 1 teaspoon of food in on top of the soil and keep the soil moist but not wet. Wrap the jar in black paper explaining that worms don't have eyes but are very sensitive to light and that in nature they only come out at night to look for food.

Note: The children could be assigned to bring in worm food before the farm is created, and each can explain what he or she brought. Live worms can be purchased at fishing supply stores.

CHAPTER 4

Activities for Children Ten to Twelve Years of Age

Cooperative Skills

1. UNTWIST

Objective

Child will use cooperative skills in a group activity.

Materials

None

Procedure

Have students stand in a tight circle, shoulder to shoulder. Instruct them to reach their right hands into the center of the circle and grab the right hand of another person. Then, instruct all to reach into the center of the circle with their left hands and grab a different person's left hand. Tell them to make sure no one has both hands of the same person. Tell the children they must work as a group to untangle the twist of persons and end up with a circle of people holding hands. The children are allowed to talk to each other, giving ideas as to how each person should move to untangle the group, but they may not let go of hands at any time.

2. NAME THAT BORDER

Objective

Child will use cooperative skills in a group activity.

Materials

☐ large map of the United States

Procedure

This is a game of working together to name states that touch each other. It requires teamwork to come up with all the answers.

Show the children the map. Discuss that maps are a great way to see which states touch each other. Explain that the group gets to look at the map for one minute, after which you will take the map away. You will then pick a state (e.g., Georgia), and the group must name all the states that touch that state.

The group must take turns providing answers so that all children have the same number of turns. If a child does not know an answer and wishes help from another student, he or she may ask for help, and another student may whisper it to him. In this way, students learn to rely on each other and build teamwork.

Incorrect answers are not penalized, as there are no points in this game. After correctly guessing all of the states that touch the first state, show the map to the group for another minute, then name another state.

> *Variation:* First-timers may have better success if only a section of the country is used at one time (e.g., cover half of the map and only use the other half to start).

3. POWER TOWER

Objective

Child will use cooperative skills in a group activity.

Materials

- ☐ recycled materials such as empty toilet paper and paper towel rolls, cardboard from pizzas, other cardboard of various shapes and sizes, plastic jars, steel vegetable cans (washed, no sharp edges), oatmeal containers
- ☐ paper clip
- ☐ plastic cup

Procedure

Place the recycled materials in a heap in the center of the circle of students. Instruct the students that, with these materials, they must build a tower as high as they can but as strong as possible. When finished, it must hold at least a paper clip on top, and if it holds the plastic cup, they are super builders! Emphasize that students must take turns adding pieces to the structure, all must get their turns, and no one can remove a piece placed by another student. Be prepared to moderate as needed throughout the activity.

4. BUILDING TEAMWORK THROUGH DISTANCE

Objective

Child will use cooperative skills in a group activity.

Materials

☐ recycled materials such as empty toilet paper and paper towel rolls, cardboard of various lengths and shapes, oatmeal containers, empty plastic peanut butter or jelly containers

☐ duct tape

☐ small vehicle

☐ tape measure

☐ pen and paper to record distances.

Procedure

Distribute the recycled materials to the group, being sure each member is given similar types and numbers of materials. Put the tape, vehicle, and tape measure in a central location where all students have access to them.

Tell the students in the group that they must use the recycled materials to build a structure that their vehicle will roll down, traveling a minimum of 3 feet. Their goal is for the vehicle to roll the farthest distance possible. Explain that they will be allowed several attempts to adjust their structures to increase the rolling distance. Offer to be the record keeper to record the distances the vehicle travels.

Emphasize that each member may only place the items he or she possesses; if a person runs out of items, or sees ways to use or place items another person possesses, he or she may suggest ways the other person may use or place the items but may not do it him- or herself. In other words, each person may only physically manipulate the items in his or her possession. However, the tape, tape measure, and vehicle may be used by all group members. Emphasize that students must use teamwork to accomplish the project. Give the group 1 minute to discuss the project before they are allowed to begin building.

5. PARQUETRY PATTERNS

Objective

Child will use cooperative skills in a group activity.

Materials

☐ multicolored parquetry blocks

☐ pattern cards

Procedure

Place a pattern on the table. Dole out the blocks needed to complete the pattern to the children. Encourage them to work together to complete the pattern. Remind them how to politely interact to complete the activity. Once completed, choose a new pattern and repeat the activity.

6. UNUSUAL CARD GAME

Objective

Child will use cooperative skills in a group activity.

Materials

- ☐ deck of cards
- ☐ thick, brightly colored marker
- ☐ several sheets of newspaper
- ☐ blackboard or easel and cardboard to keep score on
- ☐ masking tape

Procedure

Open two sheets of newspaper and lay them flat on the floor, separated from but near each other. You will have paper with four faces showing. With marker, label the four sections of the paper in large numbers: "1, 2, 3, 4." The sections of paper are to be the targets. Tape a line an appropriate distance from the paper to indicate where the "thrower" stands.

Explain to the group that this game requires teamwork. They are all on the same team, and they must take turns tossing cards on the target to gain points. If a card lands on the paper with "1," they earn one point; if it lands on the "2," they earn two points; and so forth. You keep score for them, adding up their points on the scoreboard. Tell them you will play three rounds, and each time the group must try to beat their score from the previous round.

Group members are allowed to encourage and guide each other, but all comments must be positive. All members must get equal turns. This is a great game for building teamwork.

7. NO-COOK OATMEAL COOKIES

Objective

Child will use cooperative skills in a group activity.

Materials

- ☐ ¾ cup sugar
- ☐ ⅔ cup softened butter
- ☐ 3 tablespoons cocoa
- ☐ 1 tablespoon water
- ☐ ½ teaspoon vanilla
- ☐ 2 cups dry oatmeal
- ☐ powdered sugar if desired
- ☐ large bowl
- ☐ wooden spoon
- ☐ measuring cups and spoons

Procedure

Give each child several of the ingredients. Remind them to pay attention so the ingredients can be added in the appropriate order according to the recipe. Cream the sugar and butter. Add the other ingredients except for the oatmeal and powdered sugar. Mix well. Blend in the oatmeal with the wooden spoon. Have the children roll small portions of the dough into a ball. Roll in the powdered sugar, if desired. The recipe makes 18 to 24 cookies.

The group members may offer cookies to others.

8. ICE CREAM ROLLER

Objective

Child will use cooperative skills in a group activity.

Materials

- ☐ 2 cups heavy cream
- ☐ ¾ cup sugar
- ☐ ½ cup egg substitute
- ☐ ½ teaspoon vanilla
- ☐ 1-pound coffee can
- ☐ 3–5 pound coffee can with ice
- ☐ 1 pound table salt
- ☐ rubber scraper
- ☐ bowls
- ☐ spoons

Procedure

Give each child ingredients to add and give another child responsibility for the ice and salt. Pour the first four ingredients into the smaller can and seal. Place the smaller can into the larger can surrounding the small can with the ice and salt. Seal the large can. Let the children take turns rolling the can back and forth on the floor for about half an hour. Open the cans and scrape down the side of the smaller can about every 10 minutes. Spoon the ice cream into bowls and serve. Encourage the children to invite others to enjoy their creation.

9. INSECT FARM

Objective

Child will use cooperative skills in a group activity.

Materials

- ☐ gallon jar
- ☐ soil and leaves or grass
- ☐ dark paper
- ☐ cotton soaked in water
- ☐ crumbs of bread, cookies, honey, or sugar water
- ☐ nylon netting or stocking
- ☐ rubber band

Procedure

Have the children place the soil, leaves, or grass in the jar. Find ants and place them in the jar. Cover the jar with the nylon netting or stocking and secure with the rubber band. Cover the jar with a piece of dark paper to encourage the ants to tunnel. Encourage the children to discuss how the ants work together as a team. Place the cotton in the jar for water and place the food in the jar.

Note: Ants can be ordered from science mail order companies.

10. ENERGY CHEWS

Objective

Child will use cooperative skills in a group activity.

Materials

- ☐ small cup and spoon for each child
- ☐ bowls for ingredients, ingredients for each child
- ☐ 1 tablespoon peanut butter, ½ teaspoon honey, 1 table-spoon raisins, 1 teaspoon chopped apple, 1 tablespoon dry oatmeal, measuring spoons.

Procedure

Place a copy of the recipe where each child can see it. Place the bowls with ingredients on the table. Encourage sharing of the measuring spoons and let each child place the ingredients in the cup. Mix the ingredients with the spoon and form into a ball. Chill for later or enjoy now!

Eye Contact

1. PARTNER INTERVIEWS

Objective

Child will use eye contact when speaking and listening.

Materials

None

Procedure

This activity is a fun way to practice eye contact while getting to know group members. Demonstrate what eye contact means. Describe why it is important for effective communication in both speaking and listening.

Pair each student with a partner. Instruct students to find out three interesting facts about their partners while using eye contact as they interview and answer each other. Let them know you will be observing each conversation and show them a sign you will use to cue them if they need reminders to give eye contact as they communicate.

Questions may be the same for all students (e.g., What is your middle name? Who is a famous person you admire? What is your favorite color?) or questions may be left to the students' discretion.

As students talk and listen to their partners, monitor their conversations while giving cues to increase eye contact as necessary. After all interviews are finished, allow students to introduce their partners to the whole group using eye contact as they speak. Provide cues for eye contact as needed.

2. INTRODUCE YOURSELF

Objective

Child will use eye contact when speaking and listening.

Materials

None

Procedure

Demonstrate what eye contact means. Describe why it is important for effective communication in both speaking and listening. Tell students they get to practice using eye contact while introducing themselves to the group and while listening to others introduce themselves. Let them know that you will be observing each introduction, and show them a sign you will use to cue them if they need reminders to give eye contact as they communicate.

Instruct students to think of three facts about themselves. The three facts may be defined, such as, "Tell us 3 things you like to do when you are not in school," or students may independently construct three pieces of information to share. Each group member takes a turn introducing him- or herself to the group, using eye contact while speaking. Remind listeners to give eye contact also. Provide cues as needed.

3. I'LL BE YOUR SERVER

Objective

Child will use eye contact when speaking and listening.

Materials

- ☐ refreshments (one item for each student to distribute to group)
- ☐ server's apron (optional)

Procedure

Inform students that they will each have a turn being a waiter, passing out refreshments to the rest of the group. Instruct students that good communication, including eye contact, is important to being a waiter as well as to being a consumer. Have students choose the refreshment items they will distribute. Let them take turns passing out the items, using eye contact as they ask each group member, "Would you like some _____?" Remind group members also to make eye contact as they are waited on.

4. NAME GAME

Objective

Child will use eye contact when speaking and listening.

Materials

☐ construction paper (one sheet per child)

☐ pens

Procedure

Write each student's name in capital letters down the side of a piece of paper. Give each student the paper with his or her name on it and a pen. Instruct students to think of adjectives that describe each person, but the words must begin with the letters in the person's name. Emphasize that only positive adjectives will be acceptable.

Begin with one student, telling the group to think of adjectives for him or her. Instruct students that they must use eye contact as they propose and listen to each others' ideas. While observing the activity, remind students as needed to use eye contact. Let students write the adjectives on their own papers. Encourage students to take the papers home and share with family members.

Additional Benefits: This game can be a great self-esteem builder while also provides insight into students' feelings about themselves.

5. FIND OUT—LINE UP

Objective

Child will use eye contact when speaking and listening.

Materials

None

Procedure

Explain to the group that this is a game where students get to find out information about each other and then use it to get in a line. For example, students might find out everyone's birthday and line up starting with the January birthdays at the front of the room, and the December birthdays at the back of the room.

The only rule is that, as students talk to each other to find things out, they must have eye contact with each other.

Examples of information to find out and line up accordingly include alphabetical order by first name, alphabetical order by last name, alphabetical order by name of street you live on, height; weight; how many pets you have, and so forth.

Be prepared to moderate, cueing members for eye contact as needed.

6. EXERCISES

Objective

Child will use eye contact when speaking and listening.

Materials

☐ book with exercises

Procedure

Allow the children to choose several exercises. Initially, the teacher should lead the exercises until the children can complete them independently. Remind the children that they must look at the leader to know what to do. Once the children can effectively complete the exercises, let each child take a turn in leading an exercise.

7. LET'S EAT!

Objective

Child will use eye contact when speaking and listening.

Materials

- ☐ various snack foods
- ☐ various beverages
- ☐ cups
- ☐ plates
- ☐ napkins
- ☐ utensils as needed.

Procedure

Have one child pass out the snacks. Assign another child the responsibility for the passing out the cups, plates, and so on. Remind the children that they need to look at their peers when requesting the paper products and food and beverage. Limit the amount of food and beverage given to encourage requests for more to be made with effective eye contact.

8. GET OFF MY BACK!

Objective

Child will use eye contact when speaking and listening.

Materials

☐ index cards with names of animals, objects, or other concepts

☐ adhesive tape or safety pins.

Procedure

Place a card on the back of one of the children. Let the other children see the word, but remind them that they cannot say the word out loud. The child with the card then makes eye contact with each child while asking him or her a question about the thing named on the card. Once the child guesses correctly, another child gets a turn. After each child takes a turn, the teacher can have a turn too!

9. HERE'S LOOKING AT YOU

Objective

Child will use eye contact when speaking and listening.

Materials

None

Procedure

Talk about eye contact and that it is important because people know you are talking to them. Point out that regular eye contact during a conversation lasts for about 3 to 5 seconds before people look away. Have the children take turns making eye contact for 3 to 5 seconds. Have them make eye contact for less time and for a longer time. Discuss the difference between eye contact and staring. Practice both but remind the children that staring is not always a good thing. Some people might think you are angry with them if you stare at them.

10. DON'T SAY A WORD

Objective

Child will use eye contact when speaking and listening.

Materials

- [ ] small bag or hat
- [ ] slips of paper with questions that produce a yes or no response

Procedure

Tell the children that they are going to answer the questions without talking or nodding or shaking their head. They can only show their answer by looking at the person who asked and making a face. For example, if a child really wants a new bike, the answer might be a broad smile. Demonstrate the appropriate responses if necessary.

Expressing Emotions

1. FACIAL EXPRESSION COLLAGE

Objective

Child will use facial expressions to depict emotions.

Materials

- ☐ old magazines
- ☐ scissors
- ☐ glue
- ☐ construction paper

Procedure

Label each piece of construction paper with a different emotion that you want the students to depict with facial expressions. Choose one paper and start by discussing the emotion listed on it. Talk about the feelings associated with that emotion and demonstrate accompanying facial expressions. Instruct students to look through magazines for pictures of faces depicting that emotion. Have students cut out the faces and glue them onto the paper. Have students take turns making facial expressions appropriate for each emotion before moving onto the next emotion.

2. ALPHABET EXPRESSIONS

Objective

Child will use facial expressions to depict emotions.

Materials

☐ large letters of the alphabet

☐ a mirror

Procedure

Lay out the letters of the alphabet in front of the group. Instruct children to think of a feeling they can depict with a facial expression, then pick the letter of the alphabet that feeling starts with. When all children have chosen a letter, have children go in alphabetical order making facial expressions to depict the feelings they have chosen. (Allow children to practice first in front of the mirror if they prefer.) By looking at the child's facial expressions and the beginning letter, group members try to guess the feeling the child is depicting.

3. MATCH THE WORDS TO THE FACE

Objective

Child will use facial expressions to depict emotions.

Materials

None

Procedure

The teacher makes statements with accompanying facial expressions and body language and the children have to determine if his or her words match the facial expression. Once the children are able to determine matches appropriately, the teacher can whisper a statement and facial expression to a child who can try to demonstrate it to the others. It may be very challenging for a child with AS to produce matched and mismatched statements and facial expressions.

4. WHAT MAKES ME HAPPY?

Objective

Child will use facial expressions to depict emotions.

Materials

None

Procedure

Discuss what makes some people happy. Discuss what makes each child happy. Discuss what makes them sad or not happy. Point out that some things make some people happy but not others. Discuss that it is okay for people to enjoy different things.

5. THESE ARE A FEW OF MY FAVORITE THINGS SCRAPBOOK

Objective

Child will use facial expressions to depict emotions.

Materials

- ☐ several pieces of construction paper for each child
- ☐ magazines
- ☐ two pairs of scissors
- ☐ two glue sticks
- ☐ hole punch
- ☐ string or yarn

Procedure

Discuss things that are our favorites and talk about the broad categories in which these things might fall such as foods, toys, and so forth. Label each page according to these broad categories. Look through the magazines for pictures of these things and cut them out. Glue them on the appropriate pages. When finished, punch holes in the left margin and cut string or yarn pieces to tie the pages together. Encourage sharing of the scissors and glue sticks.

6. FACES PLAY

Objective

Child will use facial expressions to depict emotions.

Materials

- ☐ paper plates
- ☐ markers
- ☐ tongue depressors
- ☐ tape

Procedure

Make plate faces depicting different emotions that can be used as hand-held masks. Facilitate the group in crafting a play that includes all the different emotions and the events that might trigger these emotions. Rehearse the play using the masks and perform it for an invited audience.

7. WHAT TO DO IF . . .

Objective

Child will use facial expressions to depict emotions.

Materials

None

Procedure

Discuss various negative scenarios that children might encounter. Scenarios might include being bullied, getting a poor grade, losing at a game, or not getting an award. Let the group determine the scenarios in which they have an interest and then problem solve as a group. It may be helpful to write down the solutions students offer. The solutions might be integrated into a social story if necessary.

8. ACT IT OUT

Objective

Child will use facial expressions to depict emotions.

Materials

☐ small bag, bowl or hat

☐ slips of paper with messages for pantomiming

Procedure

The teacher should write out a number of messages to be acted out without words. Sounds effects are fine. Each child takes a turn by picking a slip, reading the message, and acting it out. The other children try to guess the message, and the one closest to the correct answer gets to pick a slip next.

Sample Messages:

I like my new shoes.

I love to slide down the slide.

Waiting in line is no fun.

I ate too much candy and I feel sick.

I need to clean up my room.

I am late for class.

9. HELPING A FRIEND

Objective

Child will use facial expressions to depict emotions.

Materials

None

Procedure

Describe a situation in which a friend might be upset. Have the children discuss how they could go about trying to help the friend. Discuss that they should ask if the friend needs help first. If the friend says yes, then ask him or her what you can do. If the friend does not know, make some suggestions. If the friend says no, then remind the child to respect that. The child can offer to help if the friend changes his or her mind later.

10. TAKE A DEEP BREATH!

Objective

Child will use facial expressions to depict emotions.

Materials

None

Procedure

Discuss with the children what they might be able to do to relax or calm down when they are upset. Make a list of all the possible activities and then let each child make a list of those he or she prefers. Discuss why some things make one person feel better but not another. Discuss why it is okay for each person to have his or her own list of calming activities.

Turn Taking

1. TREASURE HUNT PUZZLE

Objective

Child will use turn-taking in group activities.

Materials

- ☐ poster board
- ☐ drawing or picture of a treasure chest
- ☐ glue
- ☐ pens or markers

Procedure

Draw or cut out a picture of a treasure chest (or any other treasure-like item) to glue onto a poster board. On the back of the poster, write the location where you have hidden some treat for the children. When dry, cut the treasure poster into as many pieces as you have children in the group. Label the pictures 1 through __ (number of children in group). Hide the cut poster pieces in designated areas (playground, lawn, classroom, gym, etc.).

Give each child a number corresponding to the numbers you have labeled the poster parts. Tell them you have hidden a treasure, but they must first find and assemble the pieces of the puzzle to find the treasure. Instruct the children to find a puzzle piece that matches the number you gave them. When all of the pieces are found, students take turns adding their pieces to assemble the puzzle, finally discovering where the treasure is hidden. (Don't forget to hide the treasure!) Treasure may be edible treats or small tokens.

2. BUILD A ROBOT

Objective

Child will use turn-taking in group activities.

Materials

- ☐ clean, recycled materials such as round cardboard pieces from pizzas, plastic peanut butter jars, empty toilet paper and paper towel rolls, empty steel food cans (no sharp edges), empty oatmeal boxes, plastic yogurt containers, etc.
- ☐ duct tape
- ☐ masking tape
- ☐ markers or pens

Procedure

Distribute a variety of the recycled materials to each child. Tell them that the group must build a robot, of any design they choose, but they must take turns adding pieces to construct it. Let the children discuss the construction for a while, then choose one student to begin, selecting a recycled item from his materials and declaring what robot part it constitutes. Let each of the students follow, each taping their robot parts to the first person's as they build the robot part by part. Continue until all of the parts are used or until the group declares that the robot is finished. Markers or pens may be used for adding faces or other creative features.

3. BRICK WALLS

Objective

Child will use turn-taking in group activities.

Materials

- ☐ cardboard blocks approximately the size of bricks (commercially available)
- ☐ pictures showing blocks assembled into walls of various patterns

Procedure

Distribute the blocks to students so all have the same number. Show the students a picture of a wall that they must copy; that is, they must build their wall to match the one in the picture. Students must take turns placing their blocks, and they are allowed to handle only the blocks they have been given. If a student places a block out of place according to the design, other students may suggest a better placement, point to the picture to show the difference, or otherwise verbally help the student; but they may not physically handle other students' blocks.

4. MEGA PICK-UP STICKS

Objective

Child will use turn-taking in group activities.

Materials

☐ cardboard tubes (about 3 feet long, such as those from wrapping paper) with half of the tubes painted blue, half painted red

Procedure

Divide the group into two teams, Blue and Red. Number the children on each team so they know their order for turn-taking.

Jumble the sticks up and drop them in the center of the group, just as you would with regular pick-up sticks, letting them land topsy-turvy in a heap. Flip a coin to see which team goes first. The first team tries to retrieve as many of their color tubes as they can without disturbing the positions of the other tubes. If they disturb a tube other than the one they are trying to get, it is the other team's turn. The first team to retrieve all their tubes wins. Mix the teams up for the next round so that all students will have a chance to be winners.

Variation: Have the group paint the tubes one day and play the game another day.

5. MAGNET PLAY

Objective

Child will use turn-taking in group activities.

Materials

☐ magnets

☐ objects that are attracted to magnets

☐ objects that are not attracted to magnets

Procedure

Discuss the principles of magnetism and allow the children to take turns testing what is attracted to magnets and what is not.

Variation: Drawing games that use metal flakes can be used to demonstrate the same principles. Science curricula often have units on magnets and such a unit can be used to facilitate the activity.

6. OBSTACLE COURSE WITH A REMOTE-CONTROLLED CAR

Objective

Child will use turn-taking in group activities.

Materials

- ☐ remote-controlled car
- ☐ blocks
- ☐ furniture
- ☐ items to use as obstacles and a barrier

Procedure

Set up an obstacle course for the car to navigate. Let each child take a turn practicing with the remote. Place one child on the side of the barrier so that the course is not visible. Let another child direct the movements of the car through the course. Remind the children to wait their turn and not to call out directions until it is their turn. The other children can be the spectators cheering the driver on.

7. EXPLORING SNOW

Objective

Child will use turn-taking in group activities.

Materials

- ☐ black construction paper and magnifying glass, or
- ☐ microscope and slide
- ☐ plastic bowls
- ☐ snow (freeze some in advance, if necessary)
- ☐ white paper
- ☐ two pairs of scissors

Procedure

Place the snow on the black construction paper. Allow the children to take turns examining the snow with the magnifying glass or the microscope. Discuss how the flakes look and how they differ from one another. Place snow in the bowls in various places around the room and monitor the rate at which it melts. Determine what caused faster or slower melting and discuss. Demonstrate how to fold the white paper and cut it to create snowflakes.

> *Note:* Excellent snowflake pictures are available online.

8. MAKING PLAY CLAY

Objective

Child will use turn-taking in group activities.

Materials

- ☐ large mixing bowls (metal is preferred)
- ☐ wooden spoons
- ☐ 1 cup flour
- ☐ ½ cup salt
- ☐ 6–7 tablespoons of water
- ☐ 1 tablespoon vegetable oil
- ☐ food coloring
- ☐ plastic bags or disposable storage containers
- ☐ measuring cups and spoons

Procedure

Assign each child an ingredient to add to a large mixing bowl. Slowly add water, stirring after each spoonful. Carefully add 2 to 4 drops of food coloring. Stir to distribute the color. Finish the mixing by allowing the children to use their hands. Make several colors. Let the children form different figures, sharing the different colors of clay. Store leftover clay in bags or containers.

> *Note:* The amount of water needed varies according to humidity. Figures can be placed on a cookie sheet and slowly baked at a low temperature (200 degrees) for at least 1 hour.

9. QUICK CHANGE

Objective

Child will use turn-taking in group activities.

Materials

- ☐ oversized clothing including pants, shirts, hats, gloves, belts, shoes, skirts, etc.
- ☐ stopwatch
- ☐ camera

Procedure

Have two of the children engage in a relay race putting on and taking off oversized clothing. Assign one child the job of time-keeper and choose another to serve as the starter. Other children can cheer for their peers. Shift roles until each child has served in each role. Keep the times and give awards for the fastest change, the funniest outfit, and so forth. Take photos of each child in his or her outfit.

10. BEAD STRINGING

Objective

Child will use turn-taking in group activities.

Materials

☐ decorative beads

☐ strings cut to length for necklaces and bracelets

☐ clasps

Procedure

Allow the children to select various beads to create a necklace or bracelet. Demonstrate how beads are strung and how clasps are attached.

Note: Boys may balk at bead stringing, but if a variety of beads are available in "masculine" colors, they may participate. They might be willing to participate if the end product is a gift for a family member or friend.

Topic Maintenance

1. OUTSIDE INVITATIONS

Objective

Child will use eye contact, topic maintenance, and appropriate length of communication.

Materials

Materials to put on a play, puppet show, or other group performance.

Procedure

This activity requires several sessions to plan ahead. Have the group plan a brief puppet show or some other performance. Let them practice over several sessions until they are ready to perform. Prior to the event, check with several nongroup members who are located nearby (e.g., office personnel, other instructors, janitorial crew, etc.) for permission for group members to invite them to the performance.

When the performance is ready, have students practice how they will invite the audience. Instruct students to use eye contact, stay on topic, and keep their communication to the point as they invite various people.

2. STORY CREATION

Objective

Child will use eye contact, topic maintenance, and appropriate length of communication.

Materials

None

Procedure

Explain that the group will create a story by each person adding to the information told by the previous person. The teacher begins by describing a setting and characters presumably of interest to the group. A sample beginning may start like this:

> "Early one morning on the school playground, the janitor was sweeping up trash when he noticed something shiny sticking out of the ground. He kicked at it a little and realized the shiny something was buried too deep to pull out by hand. He went to the garage and brought back a shovel, digging the dirt away to uncover the object. Very soon he was told he had a phone call, so he went inside the school to talk on the phone. Just then, the 5th grade class arrived on the playground for recess. When the kids saw the shovel and shiny object . . . "

Instruct students to pick up where the last student left off, telling part of the story for the next child to continue. Explain that you will prod them for more information if their turn is too short, or, if they talk too long, you will help them decide when their turn is finished. Help each student contribute equally to create an imaginative story. If the last child does not conclude the story, provide a story closing for the group.

3. STORY FROM OBJECTS

Objective

Child will use eye contact, topic maintenance, and appropriate length of communication.

Materials

☐ one object for each group member.

Procedure

Pass out objects to group members. Explain that the group will create a story about the objects the students now possess. Each person will add to information told by the previous person.

The teacher begins by describing a setting and inserting a few lines about an object he or she holds. Sample objects may include those that lead the children to tell a familiar story. *Example:* With a golden-haired doll, a small house, three bears, three toy chairs, three bowls and three toy beds, the group may tell "Goldilocks and the Three Bears."

Other objects may be given that lead to unique stories. Sample objects may include: a toy hammer, stuffed animals, farm set barn, toy car and driver, toy horse, jump rope, blocks of wood, and pretend food items.

Instruct students to pick up where the last student left off, telling part of a story for the next child to continue. Explain that you will prod them for more information if their turn is too short, or if they talk too long, you will help them decide when their turn is finished. Help them each contribute equally to create an imaginative story. If the last child does not conclude the story, provide a story closing for the group. Praise each member's contributions at the story's ending.

4. SPINNER TALK

Objective

Child will use eye contact, topic maintenance, and appropriate length of communication.

Materials

☐ spinner from any board game or make your own spinner.

Procedure

Choose several topics to be discussed by the group in round-robin fashion. Topic ideas include describing a dream vacation, best day of my life, what I want to be when I grow up and why, favorite subject in school and why, things I like to do with my friends, if I ruled the world this is one thing I would change, and so forth. Print the topics on paper to fit on the spinner board so that all students can take a turn spinning to determine what topic they will present.

Instruct students that they will each get a turn to spin and then present their ideas on the topic chosen by the spinner. Discuss topic maintenance and give examples of what it means to stay on topic as well as get off topic. After each child's turn, give specific feedback about the presentation, praising their on-topic statements and making brief note of portions that seemed off topic. Let students know that you found their presentations interesting.

Adaptations: Discuss how long a desired presentation should be, giving examples of presentations that are too long and detailed, too brief and lacking information, and just the right length. Explain that, if you talk too long, your audience gets bored from listening to too many details, while instilling the idea that good communication allows time for others to present their ideas as well. Give examples of effectively presenting the main points of your ideas without explaining all details at length.

---

5. STUDENT TEACHER

Objective

Child will use eye contact, topic maintenance, and appropriate length of communication.

Materials

None

Procedure

Explain to the group that, for this activity, the teacher will be the student, and the students will give feedback to the teacher regarding topic maintenance. Instruct the students to think of topics for the teacher to present. Examples may include: what I did over the weekend, how to make a peanut butter and jelly sandwich, the reasons I became a teacher, my favorite foods, games I played when I was a child, and so on. Show the students a signal (such as raising a hand or pointing a finger at you) they may use if they hear the presentation go off topic. Be sure to wander off topic as you present and respond to students signals to get back on topic.

6. ROUND-ROBIN DISCUSSION

Objective

Child will use eye contact, topic maintenance, and appropriate length of communication.

Materials

None

Procedure

Explain that a round-robin discussion is one in which each person takes a turn offering his or her ideas on a topic. Ask the group for input as to why it is important to stay on topic. If input is lacking, explain that off-topic remarks confuse listeners and detract from the point one is trying to make. Show the group a signal you will use to cue them if their remarks stray off topic.

Inform the group that today's activity is a round-robin discussion of a specific topic. An example of a topic might be: "If you lived in Florida in an area often hit by hurricanes, would you continue to live there or would you move?" Ask for a volunteer to start the round-robin, then go around the table until all students have had a chance to talk. Provide the "off-topic signal" at appropriate times during presentations. In conclusion, praise members for their interesting comments and thoughtful ideas on the topic.

7. PARACHUTE BOUNCE

Objective

Child will use eye contact, topic maintenance, and appropriate length of communication.

Materials

☐ parachute

☐ ball

Procedure

Group members gather around a parachute, holding the edges and waving it up and down. A ball is placed in the parachute, and the group is told to keep the ball on the parachute as they wave it in the air. Each time the ball falls off the parachute, the person nearest to the ball's exit point must identify a setting outside the therapy room where group members potentially can use the communication skills they have learned such as eye contact, topic maintenance, conversational turn-taking, and so forth. Settings to identify might include class presentations at school, after school events, scout meetings, church activities, and so on.

8. BALLOON SLIPS

Objective

Child will use eye contact, topic maintenance, and appropriate length of communication.

Materials

- ☐ balloons
- ☐ slips of paper to fit inside balloons
- ☐ timer

Procedure

Write the individual goals of group members on small slips of paper. Fold into small pieces and drop each into a balloon. Blow up balloons and tie to secure inflation.

Give one balloon to the group, telling them to hit it around to each other in the air until the timer beeps. Set timer for 1 minute. When timer beeps, the group must pop the balloon and read aloud the communication goal written on the slip of paper inside and explain it.

9. COMMUNICATION CHAINS

Objective

Child will use eye contact, topic maintenance, and appropriate length of communication.

Materials

- ☐ construction paper cut into strips about 4" long and ½" wide
- ☐ pens
- ☐ stapler

Procedure

Put the construction paper in the middle of the table, with the group sitting around the table. Give a pen to each student. Instruct the students to think of the communication goals they have been working on during group treatment sessions. Starting with a volunteer (or the student on your left), ask the student for one of the communication goals he or she has worked on during group. Instruct all students to write that goal on a slip of paper. Continue by asking the next person, and have students write that goal on a slip of paper. Examples of goals might be, "eye contact," "stick to the topic," "don't talk too long," and so on. If a student gets stuck and cannot think of a goal, allow others to help by offering suggestions of goals. After all students have had a turn, or after all goals have been identified, instruct students to loop the construction pieces into a chain, stapling pieces one by one to secure them. Encourage students to take the chains home to share with family.

This activity is most effective after the group has worked together for a period of time and members are somewhat familiar with the communication goals of the sessions. Colors of the paper may match a seasonal event (e.g., black and orange near Halloween, red and green near Christmas, etc.) or may be chosen by students according to their favorite colors.

10. OCCUPATION COLLAGE

Objective

Child will use eye contact, topic maintenance, and appropriate length of communication.

Materials

- ☐ magazine or catalogue pages of different people doing various jobs and of items that go along with those occupations
- ☐ butcher paper
- ☐ two glue sticks
- ☐ two pairs of scissors

Procedure

Discuss common occupations that children would come in contact with in everyday life. Talk about the jobs and what is needed to do the jobs. Provide items that might be used by a person with a certain occupation along with items not used by that person and allow discussion about what belongs and why. Glue the people and their associated items on the butcher paper. The butcher paper can be sectioned for different types of occupations (safety, education, medical, etc.).

References

Adams, L., & Earles, W. (2004, November). *Humor in children with Asperger syndrome.* Poster session presented at the annual meeting of the American Speech-Language-Hearing Association, Philadelphia, PA.

American Psychiatric Association. (1994). *Diagnostic and statistical manual of mental disorders* (4th ed.). Washington, DC: Author.

Attwood, T. (1998). *Asperger's syndrome: A guide for parents and professionals.* Philadelphia, PA: Jessica Kingsley Publishers.

Baron-Cohen, S. (1990). Autism: A specific cognitive disorder of "mind-blindness." *International Review of Psychiatry, 2,* 81–90.

Baron-Cohen, S., O'Riordan, M., Stone, V., Jones, R., & Plaisted, K. (1999). Recognition of faux pas by normally developing children and children with Asperger syndrome or high-functioning autism. *Journal of Autism and Developmental Disorders, 29*(5), 407–418.

Blankenship, K. (2000). *Theory of mind and children with learning disabilities.* Unpublished master's thesis, Radford University, Radford, VA.

Bosacki, S. L. (2000). Theory of mind and self-concept in preadolescents: Links with gender and language. *Journal of Educational Psychology, 92*(4), 709–717.

Cumine, V., Leach, J., & Stevenson, G. (1998). *Asperger syndrome: A practical guide for teachers.* London: David Fulton.

Earles, W. (2003). *Perception of and response to humor in children with Asperger syndrome.* Unpublished manuscript.

Ehlers, S., & Gillberg, C. (1993). The epidemiology of Asperger syndrome: a total population study. *Journal of Child Psychology and Psychiatry, 43,* 1327–1350.

Frith, U. (1989). *Autism: Explaining the enigma.* Oxford, England: Blackwell.

Gilberg, C., & Gilberg, I. C. (1989). Asperger syndrome—some epidemiological considerations: A research note. *Journal of Child Psychology and Psychiatry, 30,* 631–638.

Jones, G. (2005). Executive function. In J. Neisworth & P. Wolfe (Eds.), *The autism encyclopedia* (p. 75). Baltimore: Paul H. Brookes.

Landers, E. (2005). Self-regulation. In J. Neisworth & P. Wolfe (Eds.), *The autism encyclopedia* (pp. 184–185). Baltimore: Paul H. Brookes.

Loftin, R. (2005). Self-management interventions. In J. Neisworth & P. Wolfe (Eds.), *The autism encyclopedia* (p. 184). Baltimore: Paul H. Brookes.

Lord-Laron, V., & Kaufman, N. (2005, March). *Asperger syndrome.* Paper presented at the Health Education Symposium, Chapel Hill, NC.

Majjiviona, J., & Prior, M. (1995). Comparison of Asperger's syndrome and high-functioning autistic children on a test of motor impairment. *Journal of Autism and Developmental Disorders, 25,* 23–39.

Moyes, R. (2003). *I need help with school! A guide for parents of children with autism and Asperger syndrome.* Arlington, TX: Future Horizons, Inc.

National Institute on Deafness and Other Communication Disorders. (n.d.). *Autism and communication.* Retrieved December 16, 2004 from http://www.nidcd.nih.gov/health/voice/autism.asp

Neisworth, J., & Wolfe, P. (2005). *The autism encyclopedia.* Baltimore: Paul H. Brookes.

Roffey, S., Tarrant, T., & Majors, K. (1994). *Young friends.* London: Cassell Publishing.

Vuletic, L. (2005). Sensory processing. In J. Neisworth & P. Wolfe (Eds.), *The autism encyclopedia* (pp. 187–188). Baltimore: Paul H. Brookes.

Watters, A. (2005). *Theory of mind and children with Asperger syndrome.* Unpublished master's thesis, Radford University, Radford, VA.

Wing, L., & Gould, J. (1979). Severe impairments of social interaction and associated abnormalities in children: Epidemiology and classification. *Journal of Autism and Childhood Schizophrenia, 9,* 11–29.

Yeargin-Allsopp, M., Rice, C., Karapurkar, T., Doernberg, N., Boyle, C., & Murphy, C. (2003). Prevalence of autism in a US metropolitan area. *Journal of the American Medical Association, 289*(1), 49–55.

APPENDIX A

Checklist for Instructors on the Go

The following is a list of the materials used most often in this activity manual. These items could be kept in a large box for transportation from setting to setting.

☐ Paper plates
☐ Construction paper
☐ Yarn
☐ Magazines
☐ Tape
☐ Scissors
☐ Markers
☐ Cotton balls
☐ Paints
☐ Paper cups

☐ String
☐ Pencils
☐ Crayons
☐ Paper towels
☐ Shower curtain liner
  (or drop cloth)
☐ Straws
☐ Butcher paper
☐ Cookie cutters

APPENDIX B

Activities That Need No Materials

The following activities require no materials for implementation.

Cats on the Fence
Eye to Eye, People to People
Find Out—Line Up
Follow the Leader
Helping a Friend
Here's Looking at You
How Do I Move?
How Do You Do?
If You Are Happy and You
    Know It!
Introduce Yourself
Match the Words to the Face
    Partner Interviews

Read My Face
Red Light, Green Light
Round-Robin Discussion
Stop, Drop, and Roll
Story Creation
Student Teacher
Take a Deep Breath!
Teddy Bear Song
Untwist
Watch the Leader
What Makes Me Happy?
What to Do If . . .

Alphabetical Index

Thematic Index

Problem Solving and Team Building

Seasons and Holidays